Evaluation in
Occupational Health Practice

Evaluation in
Occupational Health Practice

Editors

Ewa Menckel
MSc, PhD
and
Peter Westerholm
MD FFOM

with a Foreword by Jean-François Caillard

INTERNATIONAL COMMISSION
ON OCCUPATIONAL HEALTH - ICOH

COMMISSION INTERNATIONALE
DE LA SANTE AU TRAVAIL - CIST

Founded in 1906 as Permanent Commission

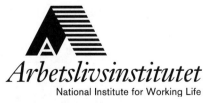

Arbetslivsinstitutet
National Institute for Working Life

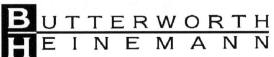

Butterworth-Heinemann
Linacre House, Jordan Hill, Oxford OX2 8DP
225 Wildwood Avenue, Woburn, MA 01801-2041
A division of Reed Educational and Professional Publishing Ltd

℞ A member of the Reed Elsevier plc group

OXFORD AUCKLAND BOSTON JOHANNESBURG
MELBOURNE NEW DELHI

First published 1999

British Library Cataloguing in Publication Data
A catalogue record for this book is available from the British Library

Library of Congress Cataloguing in Publication Data
A catalogue record for this book is available from the Library of Congress

ISBN 0 7506 4303 X

Typeset by Keytec Typesetting Ltd, Bridport, Dorset, UK
Printed and bound in Great Britain by Biddles Ltd, Guildford and King's Lynn

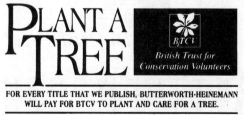

FOR EVERY TITLE THAT WE PUBLISH, BUTTERWORTH-HEINEMANN
WILL PAY FOR BTCV TO PLANT AND CARE FOR A TREE.

Contents

Contributors

Editors

Ewa Menckel, MSc, PhD, is Associate Professor of Work Science and a specialist in the psychology of work at the National Institute for Working Life, Sweden. She received her doctorate concerning occupational health services from the Department of Public Health Sciences at Karolinska Institute. Her research areas are: workplace health and safety issues, occupational injury prevention, and the development of models and methods for intervention and evaluation. She is responsible in Sweden for the EU programme 'Workplace Health Promotion'.

Peter Westerholm, MD, FFOM, is Professor of Occupational Epidemiology at the National Institute for Working Life, Sweden. He has been Chairman of the ICOH Scientific Committee for Health Services Research and Evaluation in Occupational Health since 1993. He is responsible for postgraduate training of occupational health physicians in Sweden and his research interests include psychological and social determinants of occupational health and epidemiology of occupationally related cancer and cardiovascular disease.

Editorial board

Ewa Menckel, Peter Westerholm, Nico Plomp, Jos Verbeek, Kaj Husman, Johann Behrens, Stuart Whitaker

Contributors

Raymond Agius, MD, FRCP (Lond. & Edin.), FFOM, is a senior lecturer in Occupational and Environmental Health at the University of Edinburgh, UK, and a consultant in Occupational Medicine at the Royal Infirmary of Edinburgh. His research interests have included quality and audit, occupational stress, and occupational and environmental respiratory ill-health. He is a Past-President of the British Occupational Hygiene Society.

Nicholas A. Ashford, PhD, JD, is Professor of Technology and Policy at MIT and adjunct faculty at the Harvard and Boston University Schools of Public Health. His books include *Crisis in the Workplace, Monitoring the Worker for Exposure and Disease,* and *Technology, Law, and the Working*

Environment. He is a Fellow of the American Association for the Advancement of Science and an adviser to the United Nations Environment Program.

Johann Behrens, Prof. Dr phil, has been chairperson of the ISIS-Institute in Frankfurt am Main, Germany since 1982. In 1994 he was active in establishing the Department of Occupational Medicine, Public Health and Health System Research of the University of Bremen. He served as prodean of the Faculty of Health and Nursing Sciences of the University of Applied Sciences, Fulda from 1995 to 1998. He has served as director of the Institute (School) of Health and Nursing Sciences of the Martin Luther University in Halle since 1998.

Diane Berthelette earned her PhD in Public Health from the Université de Montréal, Canada. Since 1989, Dr Berthelette has been a staff member in the School of Business Administration at the Université du Québec à Montréal, where she performs Evaluative Research in Occupational Health and Safety. In addition she is a member of the university's Groupe de recherche interdisciplinaire en santé.

Kathleen Brown, RN, PhD, is a Professor in the University of Alabama School of Nursing Graduate Programs, USA, and Co-Principal Investigator of the City of Birmingham Good Health Program.

Kerstin Ekberg has a degree in psychology and gained her PhD in medicine at the Linköping University, Sweden. During the past decade her research has mainly involved epidemiological studies on musculoskeletal disorders and evaluation of rehabilitation of disorders in the neck and shoulders. She is now a professor in rehabilitation of work-related disorders and human resources development.

Gillian Fletcher, MB, ChB, FRCP, MFOM, was a clinical research fellow in the Department of Public Health Sciences University of Edinburgh, UK, and is now a consultant in occupational medicine with Fife Healthcare NHS Trust.

James Hilyer, MPH, Ed. D, is an Assistant Professor in the Division of Preventive Medicine, University of Alabama at Birmingham School of Medicine, and is Director of the City of Birmingham Fitness Center, USA.

Carel Hulshof, MD, PhD, is an occupational physician and a senior lecturer at the Coronel Institute, Amsterdam, The Netherlands. He is especially interested in the evaluation of occupational health programmes. He developed and evaluated a prevention programme on the adverse effects of whole-body vibration. He coordinates a national programme on the development of guidelines for occupational health.

Kaj Husman, MD, PhD (University of Helsinki, Finland), gained an MSc in Health Services Planning and Epidemiology at the University of

British Columbia, Canada, in 1983 and became Professor in Occupational Medicine at the University of Kuopio, Finland, in 1985. His current position is Head of the Department of Occupational Medicine and the Research and Development Centre for OHS, at the Finnish Institute of Occupational Health.

Karl Kuhn, Dr, MA, is Director and Professor and Head of the 'Social and Economic Affairs' Group at the Federal Institute for Occupational Health and Safety in Dortmund, Germany. His research interests include: studies in work organization; monitoring of working conditions; causes of premature incapacity to work; stress and analysis of psychosocial workload; economics of OSH; and workplace health promotion. He is Project Leader of the European Network of Workplace Health Promotion and Head of Studies in Social Sciences at the universities of Tubingen, Germany, and Lund and Stockholm, Sweden.

Matti Lamberg, MD, DPH, is a specialist in general and occupational medicine. He worked in primary health care from 1970 to 1977. He served for six years in health administration in the Finnish Ministry of Justice until 1983, and then in the National Board of Health and the Ministry of Social Affairs and Health. He is responsible for administration of occupational health services in Finland, including the preparation of legislation. He has done development work and published in the field of health policy, health care administration and quality management in occupational health.

Robert Lee, BSC, MSC, is a Research Associate in the Medical Statistics Unit at the University of Edinburgh, UK. He has been employed as a statistician in the MSU since 1990 and has been involved in a variety of collaborative research projects with clinicians from both within and outside the university.

Terje Lie, Cand. polit., is a Senior Researcher at RF–Rogaland Research, Norway, and coordinator for work environment and health since 1982. Areas of specialization are health services, evaluation studies, social impact analysis, work environment, work and family, etc. He has published on health and social services, work environment and other topics, and teaches in sociology and welfare policy.

Takashi Muto, MD, is an Associate Professor in the Department of Public Health, Juntendo University School of Medicine, Japan. He received his doctorate in medicine from Keio University. His research focuses on evaluation of occupational health services. He has published *Evaluation of Health Promotion and Education* and *Method for the Economic Evaluation of Health Programmes* (in Japanese).

John Øvretveit, PhD, MIHSM, is Professor of Health Policy and Management at the Nordic School of Public Health in Gothenburg, Sweden and Director of the Postgraduate Diploma training in health care quality at

Bergen University School of Medicine, where he is an Associate Professor. Previously he worked as a clinician in the British NHS and then as director of the Health Services Centre, Brunel University, UK. He undertakes health management teaching, research and consultancy, evaluation projects, and has published widely on the subjects of health service quality, interprofessional cooperation and health reforms.

Jorma Rantanen, MD, Dr Med Sci, is Director General of the Finnish Institute of Occupational Health, with a scientific emphasis primarily in occupational health disciplines but also in medical biochemistry, radiation biology and toxicology. He has authored or co-authored more than 300 research reports, book chapters and books. During the past decade his published works have focused on implications of technological change and information technology with regard to occupational health and evaluations of effects and cost-efficiency of occupational health interventions.

Kathleen Rest, PhD, MPA, is Associate Professor of Occupational and Environmental Health at the University of Massachusetts Medical Center. Her research interests are US and international occupational and environmental health policy and education. Her publications address workers' compensation, surveillance of occupational illness, worker participation, and ethics. Dr Rest is chairperson of the US National Advisory Committee on Occupational Safety and Health.

Joanna Uttley, MA, MB, ChB, D.Obst., DFOM, is a part-time occupational health physician with experience in various occupational health centres in Scotland, UK, mainly dealing with health care workers.

Willeke van der Weide, PhD, is a human movement scientist who recently wrote a thesis on the quality of occupational rehabilitation of patients with low back pain. She is currently working at the TNO-institute on a project on implementation of quality systems in hospitals.

Jos Verbeek, MD, PhD, is an occupational physician teaching and researching occupational health at the Coronel Institute, Amsterdam, The Netherlands. His special interest is occupational rehabilitation by occupational physicians of workers with low back pain. He works part-time as an occupational physician at the Occupational Health Service in Amsterdam.

Axel Wannag, MD, has been a Senior Adviser to the Norwegian Labour Inspectorate since 1994. He joined occupational medicine in 1971 as a student and researcher in industrial toxicology and entered the occupational health service in 1977 as an occupational physician. From 1987 to 1991 he studied structure and activity within the Norwegian occupational health service. He is a provisional adviser to WHO.

Michael Weaver, RN, PhD, is an Associate Professor in the University of

Alabama School of Nursing Graduate Programs, USA, and is Principal Investigator of the City of Birmingham Good Health Program.

Stuart Whitaker, PhD, M Med Sc, OHNC, RGN, RMN, MIOSH Research Fellow at the University of Birmingham, is Honorary Lecturer in Health Sciences at the University of Wolverhampton and Chair of the UK Occupational Health Nurses Research Forum. He is a WHO Consultant. He has been involved in evaluation of occupational health practice since 1990. He has been a member of the ICOH scientific committee on Health Services Research since 1992. His current research is into sickness absence, pre-employment assessment and fitness to work. He has an interest in ethics and social policy in relation to occupational health care.

Foreword

by Jean-François Caillard
President of the International Commission on Occupational Health

The publication of this book is a very important event for all of us as occupational health professionals, and also for all those who have responsibility for the elaboration and implementation of means to protect the health of working men and women. For it helps us answer two questions: what has been achieved in the field of occupational health since the description, almost 4000 years ago, of one of the first occupational injuries – by Imothep, the Egyptian physician – and what will be achieved tomorrow?

Acquisition of knowledge on the relations between work and human health has been constantly in progress. Tools and methods for prevention have been conceived. Since the second part of the nineteenth century, in many countries at least, regulations and agreements have been formulated to prevent the effects of occupational hazards and maintain workers' health at the highest possible level.

As we approach the twenty-first century, 120 million occupational accidents and between 68 and 157 million diseases associated with work are registered in the world each year. According to WHO, only 20–50% of workers have access to occupational health services in industrialized countries. The figure is less than 10% elsewhere.

Anyone contemplating the future of occupational health policies is immediately confronted with a string of key questions. Among the most important are those concerned with the evolution of the workforce throughout the world, the consequences for human health of new hazards and new forms of work organization, the impact of intensifying economic competition, and the relation between occupational and environmental health.

But today, one set of questions overshadows all others. How are strategies to be defined and implemented to reach our goal of occupational health and well-being? What are the best means available to achieve this goal? How do we access the resources required? How can occupational health services be offered not only to a minority, but to all workers in the world?

Whether it be at national, regional or global level, the final responsibility for answering these questions rests on representatives of the parties involved – workers and employers – and on the various kinds of officers entrusted with health and labour policies. But occupational health professionals, because of their unique capacity to appraise the reality of the problems that have to be solved, also have great responsibility for how these questions are answered. They have to develop new tools – in particular those of evaluation – and acquire new habits and ways of working.

The various chapters in this book have been written to help occupational health professionals in this task. Scientific approaches, pragmatic case studies, and ethical and economic considerations are all presented with a clarity that is infused by the authors' enthusiasm. Each contributor has considerable experience of his or her national practice within the arena. This has been gathered together within the Scientific Committee on Health Services Research and Evaluation in Occupational Health of the International Commission on Occupational Health.

Evaluation, a step that has not been natural for physicians and other specialists in occupational health up to now, and its corollary, strategic research, are sources of great intellectual satisfaction. They are tools of conviction for those who, on several counts, are interested in public health and the good running of enterprises.

The consequences of utilizing such tools are not only greater efficiency on the part of occupational health services in terms of better output, improved valuation and enhanced quality. They also nourish ethical thought on man's place in modern systems of production, and help promote the essential value represented by workers' health throughout the world.

The appearance of this book, the first on this important topic, is a landmark event. I am particularly pleased to welcome it on behalf of the International Commission on Occupational Health, and to thank its editors and authors for making the results of their research and thought available to us all.

Acknowledgements

The preparation of this textbook has been a challenging task, made possible only through the combined efforts of a number of individuals.

As editors, we would first like to give our thanks to the editorial board that took the initiative for the writing of the book. The board offered support throughout its development, both sketching out an outline and discussing detailed contents. We also express our sincere appreciation of all the contributors for their hard work and dedication in producing their manuscripts, and for cooperation shown in relation to deadlines.

A special word of thanks goes to Jon Kimber for the great amount of effort he put into the manuscripts as a language editor and for putting them together in consistent shape. Thanks also to Gunilla Sanegård for technical editing of the manuscript and for help with the whole editing process. We also acknowledge the work of experienced science journalist Benny Kullinger, for his valuable ideas on the book and its layout.

Ewa Menckel and Peter Westerholm

Glossary

ACOEM	American College of Occupational and Environmental Medicine
CBA	cost–benefit analysis
CEA	cost-effectiveness analysis
DALYs	Disability Adjusted Life Years
COHS	Commission of Occupational Health and Safety
FIOH	Finnish Institute of Occupational Health
GOHSP	Good Occupational Health Service Practice
HSR	health services research
ICOH	International Commission on Occupational Health
ILO	International Labour Office
ISO	International Standards Organization
MSEs	medium-sized enterprises
NIOH	National Institute of Occupational Health (US)
NIVA	Nordic Institute for Advanced Training in Occupational Health
OHP	occupational health programme
OHS	occupational health services
RCT	randomized controlled trial
SMEs	small and medium-sized enterprises
SSEs	small-scale enterprises
WHO	World Health Organization

Part 1
EVALUATION APPROACHES AND MODELS

Introduction and objectives

Ewa Menckel and Peter Westerholm

This book addresses the principles and issues involved in evaluating occupational health practice. Particular attention is paid to the role played by occupational health services (OHS). Our aim has been to provide an introductory textbook and easy-to-read guide to good OHS evaluation. It is hoped that this will lead to good management of services, enhancement of performance standards and increased utility of the services rendered. We have assembled an international group of authors in the occupational health field who have a wide range of experiences and insights in this broad, multidisciplinary domain. This provides a good basis for obtaining comprehensive coverage of the many issues involved.

This first chapter is introductory by nature. It states the rationale for the book, and highlights the importance of adopting an evaluative approach to the provision of OHS, and to developing performance, effectiveness and efficiency in occupational health practice. The target groups of the book are defined, and readers' attention is drawn to the specific features of occupational health that distinguish it from primary health care. The ultimate goals of health service evaluations are emphasized.

Evaluation in an OHS context

Most people concerned with health services perform evaluations in their everyday work. This book is about evaluation of work-related health activities, with particular attention paid to work in OHS. It is written primarily to meet the needs of people who, in their roles in OHS, in other health services or in enterprises, become involved in issues of evaluation of performance or quality. They may be providers, purchasers or consumers of OHS. For example, the need to perform evaluations may arise in exercising management responsibilities in health service organizations. Professionals in occupational health perform evaluations in the course of carrying out their work, just as other professionals do. Evaluating is an integral part of a professional role. The idea is to gauge one's performance against an ideal, or at least in relation to a standard perceived as a benchmark. The process may be more or less conscious. It applies to all the planning, task performance and responsibilities of OHS.

Most commonly, evaluative approaches have been restricted to examining selected items in services or service operations. For example, the health status and health characteristics of personnel in customer enterprises are assessed, as too are hazards and other conditions in the workplace. This may be done in a more or less formalized manner. There are also large differences between evaluations with regard to approaches and methods used.

Evaluations of providers of services are much less frequently practised. This is in itself a cause of concern. In a world increasingly aware of the importance of product and performance quality, and one that treats customers' needs and demands as a fundamental basis for all activities, evaluations of health service performance assume critical importance. We can safely predict that evaluations of OHS will be increasingly implemented in the future.

It is important here to add that occupational health professionals and practitioners of occupational medicine, managers of health services and even policymakers and advisers in enterprises or in government service are usually not trained or otherwise equipped to perform formal evaluations. Accordingly, this book is in part designed for use as a basic introductory textbook.

There are indications that the first decade of the next millennium will place severe strains on health service organizations and systems throughout the world. Rising demands from the public will have to be met with shrinking resources and under constant pressure for cost containment. Despite this, the systems will still have to be responsive to the needs of the individuals and populations served. Freedom of choice for customers is a quality feature that is assuming increasing importance. This development can be observed both in public health service systems and organizations, and in the private sector, where OHS operates in most countries.

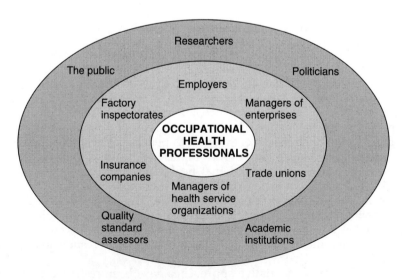

Figure 1.1 *Target groups for OHS evaluation*

This book is concerned with the arena of occupational health. The field has certain characteristics that distinguish it from general health services and primary health care systems. One of these is the central significance of a direct relationship with the customer/client. The active participation of the customer is of prime importance in all occupational health practice and, accordingly, in evaluations addressing issues related to such practice.

Other distinctive features are:

- OHS clients and providers may have differing views with regard to service needs and priorities in the planning and provision of services;
- service delivery is highly professionalized, implying that poor quality or performance is not immediately obvious to clients and service consumers;
- the complex provider–client relationship entails that the satisfaction of needs of many stakeholders (including individual employees, groups of employees, employers, management, health professionals, insurance bodies, government agencies) has to be striven for.

OHS professionals carry out their tasks in a setting and context that has undergone radical changes over the past decades. There is ongoing globalization of economies and markets, increasing transnational collaboration and networking, constant development of production technologies, and enhanced dependence on informatics and telecommunications. The panorama of occupational health risks has changed drastically. The pursuit of quality has become one of the dominant features of all production, including production of services. During the 1990s the health sector has been influenced by this trend, which has obvious implications for evaluation.

This book aims to provide an overview of the concepts, principles and issues related to evaluations of OHS. There are many ideas and approaches involved in evaluations of health services, each involving issues of objectives, procedures and methodologies. These have to be resolved and reconciled with the underlying questions and the ultimate purpose of evaluation.

The primary target group of this book consists of occupational health professionals. This broad category includes occupational health physicians and nurses, physiotherapists and ergonomists, occupational hygienists, safety engineers, occupational psychologists and managers of OHS units or organizations. We give high priority to those in these roles, with a view to facilitating their self-evaluation, implementation of benchmarking procedures, participation in formal auditing procedures and peer review of service performance and standards. The book has also been written with an eye to the needs of all those who purchase and use OHS – the customers and clients, who have a legitimate interest in seeking a service of adequate quality and cost-effectiveness, while at the same time requiring that ethical standards are satisfied. Further, although the book does not specifically address the interests and needs of health service researchers, we hope it will provide useful reading for such specialists. Our target groups can thus be positioned within three concentric circles, as shown in Figure 1.1.

OHS are human-service organizations in modern society which have been explicitly designed to manage and promote the safety, health and welfare of citizens at work. According to Hasenfeld (1983), human-service organizations have two distinct key characteristics. First, they work directly with and impact on people, whose attributes and conditions of life they attempt to shape. Secondly, they are mandated to protect and to promote the welfare of the people they serve. Indeed, this is what justifies their existence.

According to Rossi (1978), assessment of performance in human-service organizations typically involves probing of the following questions:

- Is the organization reaching its target population?
- Is it providing its mandated services?
- Are the services effective?
- Are the services provided efficiently?

In recent years, although many efforts have been made to assess performance of different human-service organizations, results have been generally dismal. More often than not, the outcome has been a failure to demonstrate programme effectiveness and efficiency. As Rossi (1978) puts it, 'Most programmes, when properly evaluated, turn out to be ineffective or at best marginally accomplishing their set aims. There are several possible explanations for this. First, the objectives of the organizations evaluated may have been multiple and difficult to summarize in simple performance criteria. Second, the nature of the service technology precludes accurate measurement. Third, isolating effects of services from extraneous factors is exceedingly difficult. Fourth, effects of services on clients are not readily quantifiable.' That the results of assessments are seldom unequivocal, and therefore open to many interpretations, has been emphasized by Hasenfeld (1983).

The book addresses all these issues. Contributions in the first section of the book deal with the 'bread and butter' of the subject – explaining the theoretical basis, concepts and methodology of evaluation. The second section consists of case studies and project descriptions, supplied by authors from a variety of countries, which focus on specific questions and highlight issues of evaluation in a contextual setting. A third and concluding section highlights some important ethical and economical perspectives and the implication for evaluations of occupational health and safety management of current developments in labour markets and work organization.

In a multi-authored book of this kind some degree of overlapping of content is difficult to avoid. But, in our view, total alignment should not even be sought. The ultimate objective of evaluation is to provide a basis for development. A prerequisite for this is that the principles of central importance in implementing evaluations in occupational health are adhered to. These, in our experience, are best understood when described in different contextual settings. We have kept this idea constantly in mind during the editing process.

It is the Editors' hope that readers will find within these pages enjoyable reading as well as food for thought and reflection.

References

Hasenfeld, Y. (1983) *Human Service Organizations.* Englewood Cliffs, NJ: Prentice–Hall.

Rossi, P.H. (1978) Some issues in the evaluation of human services delivery. In: *The Management of Human Services* (R.C. Sarri and Y. Hasenfeld, eds). New York: Columbia University Press, pp. 235–61.

2

General principles and implementation in OHS evaluation

Kaj Husman

Evaluation of occupational health services (OHS) is not only an interesting research field, but has become an essential practical tool for service providers to develop such services – to evaluate means and effect change. We have to define the objectives and content of OHS in practice before any actual evaluation is performed, and also to establish who is the client for evaluation. A variety of methods can be used for the evaluation of OHS. Here, the systems model is described in detail. The development process of the national farmers' OHS system in Finland is used as an example of how the model is applied in a quasi-experimental design. Emphasis is placed on the importance of process as well as outcome indicators.

Reasons for OHS evaluation

For many reasons, the evaluation of occupational health services (OHS) is now more important than it has ever been. OHS are facing new challenges due to rapid changes in working life and the work environment. At the same time, new discoveries and technological advances have made it possible to broaden the preventive and curative activities of OHS – but only at a price. We have to decide what to do with the resources we have, which entails prioritizing, and therefore creates an *internal* need for evaluation. On the other hand, economic recession has threatened OHS with cutbacks. We have to justify the existence of OHS to its financiers, which gives rise to an *external* need for evaluation. In order to establish a firm basis for developing occupational health services, their inputs, processes, outputs, outcomes and impacts need to be evaluated in the light of both general and specific objectives.

Objectives of OHS

Evaluation of health care can be defined as 'the assessment of effectiveness, efficiency, acceptability and acceptance of a health care system or programme in achieving the stated objectives'. This is the definition formulated by WHO in 1982. At the outset, we have to identify the objectives of the activity that we are going to evaluate. Both the planning and evaluation of OHS should serve the objectives of those services themselves. These vary according to the degree of industrialization and development in a country, the level of other (primary) health care services and the ideological (political) bases and specific legislation concerning OHS safety policy in each country.

Looking at the recommendations proffered by WHO and the ILO, the overall objectives of OHS can be regarded as being embodied in five principles. The terminology is derived from that used to discuss the targets of 'Health for All by the Year 2000':

- protect workers against hazards at work (the protection and prevention principle);
- adapt work and the work environment to the capabilities of workers (the adaptation principle);
- enhance the physical, mental and social well-being of workers (the workplace health-promotion principle);
- minimize the consequences of occupational hazards (accidents and injuries) and occupational and work-related diseases (the cure and rehabilitation principle);
- provide general health care services for workers and their families, both curative and preventive, in the workplace from nearby facilities (the general primary health care principle).

As an example of the implementation of these principles, we explore the development of OHS in Finland. Observers from many other countries may note similarities with their own system. The most recent statement of OHS objectives in Finland is contained in a decision of the Council of State from 1995. The objectives of what is called 'Good OHS Practice' are:

- a healthy and safe working environment;
- a well-functioning work community;
- the prevention of work-related diseases;
- the maintenance and promotion of employees' working and functioning capacities.

These objectives can be achieved by improving the work environment and work community (i.e. psychosocial factors), and by influencing individuals at the work site (both employers and employees).

Occupational health services in Finland have their origins in the curative services provided by employers' medical stations at the beginning of the twentieth century. The services were organized because there was no public health care. Further, since the population was not wealthy enough to buy medical care, the private market was almost non-existent. At that time, social welfare and health care were almost entirely the responsibility of employers, and existed almost only in quite large industrial enterprises.

But, over nearly a century of OHS practice, new objectives have come to the fore. The prevention of work-related diseases after the Second World War, the prevention of public health problems in the 1970s, and – more recently – an emphasis on working ability and lifestyle have broadened the scope of OHS in Finland and many other developed countries.

This shift in content of OHS reflects the move away from their being conceived as in the interest solely of employers and reliant on employer philanthropy. More broadly, it is now in society's interest to have a population – especially a working population – that is healthy and in good condition. The time perspective of OHS activities has also changed, for example, with regard to those directed at individual employees. The provision of immediate medical care provided close to the work site has been superseded – first by risk-oriented preventive and curative activities, later by an emphasis on client relations and overall lifetime well-being. Health and well-being is now taken into consideration not only during the economically active years but also during retirement.

The variety of activities within OHS can be grouped into four broad categories according to the various interests to which they are related:

- prevention of work-related diseases and injuries at the individual level (e.g. through health examinations);
- improvement of work conditions (e.g. through work site visits or lectures);
- prevention of public health problems related to lifestyle (such as elevated cholesterol, smoking, and a sedentary way of life);
- curative activities.

There is wide variation in the objectives of OHS organizations between different international organizations and different countries.

The ILO definition of OHS emphasizes the prevention of work-related aspects of ill-health, while the WHO definition includes health promotion activities of a general nature, e.g. cholesterol lowering, hypertension control, smoking cessation and fitness. Based on which objectives are considered, there is, of course, variation in the content of OHS.

Maybe, however, we can agree that OHS encompass certain core activities. A list might cover workplace surveillance and assessment of work-related health hazards – risk evaluation; information and education of employees on hazards; management consultation; pre-employment examinations; periodic occupational health examinations; consulting hours (including curative care); occupational rehabilitation/maintaining work ability; and maintaining a first-aid organization. In The Netherlands and Finland, for example, provision of such activities is obligatory under national legislation.

Van Dijk and colleagues (1993) define such instruments as 'circumscript and formalized working methods and measurement protocols, inclusive equipment and strategies'. And, as pointed out in Hulshof *et al.* (1998), they may be the subjects of OHS evaluation studies in themselves. The idea is that the quality of OHS can be enhanced when applied instruments are judged and improved.

Principles of OHS evaluation

Evaluation of OHS belongs to the domain of health services research (HSR). HSR involves the systematic investigation and evaluation of health services in terms of their inter-relationship with all health-related factors, and with such measures as feasibility, need, coverage, effectiveness, utilization, cost and efficiency. HSR is multidisciplinary and ideally should result in the improvement of the decision-making process and the optimization of resource use. This definition can be applied to the evaluation of an OHS system.

There are specific criteria for measuring the success of health programmes. Evidence is collected systematically from a representative sample of units under study. Usually, evidence is translated into quantitative measures (e.g. OHS in Finland cover 90% of the employees), and then compared with a criteria set (e.g. OHS should cover 100% of Finnish employees). Conclusions are then drawn about the merits of the system under study. Evaluation of an OHS system gives a firm basis for its further development, whether this entails enlarging the target system or cutting it back.

The evaluation research process is more expensive and time-consuming than making off-hand estimates that rely merely on intuition, opinion, or trained sensibility. But it provides a rigour that is particularly important when:

- the outcomes to be evaluated are complex, difficult to investigate, or made up of numerous elements reacting in diverse ways;
- the decisions to be made are important and expensive;
- evidence is needed to convince others about the validity of previous conclusions drawn;
- there is a need to improve the quality of the services.

Most health care programmes are set up without prior evaluation. But, usually, they are much easier to evaluate than other social programmes – because, on the whole, they have clear-cut, specific goals. This remains true despite the fact that performance of evaluation in the sector has often been opposed on the grounds that outcomes of health services cannot be measured, or are difficult to measure.

Different levels – different viewpoints

The application of HSR concepts and methods to the evaluation of OHS is a relatively new field of scientific enquiry. In this context, evaluation research means the evaluation of an OHS system at different levels and from different viewpoints. The same principles are applicable in both evaluation and the ongoing development undertaken by OHS staff themselves, and also in quality assurance or continuous quality improvement.

The first step is to establish why, for which client, and in whose interest, evaluation research is to be performed. The various interest groups or stakeholders have been classified by Menckel (1993) into five groups according to evaluation level:

- **the government or the community**, which might wish to assess the contribution made by OHS to health work in general, and whether such activities follow accepted norms, directives, laws;
- **the owners of OHS (and the trade union organizations or any other party),** who might wish to assess how their financial investments have been utilized (or whether others should be contemplated), how well contractual agreements have been kept, and how effective the work has been;
- **the clients of OHS (company management, supervisory staff or employers)**, who might wish to offer their views on efforts made so far, and who might participate in the planning of activities for the future;
- **OHS management**, who might wish to evaluate operations as a whole, encompassing anything from the benefits provided to clients to operative efficiency;
- **professional practitioners within OHS**, who might wish to follow up particular methods and their own activities to see whether desired effects have been achieved.

We have to be clear about the use of any particular evaluation and who the client of the evaluation is. Is it the owners of OHS or the providers of the services? These questions relate to the question of who is doing the evaluation. Can it be done by OHS personnel or should it be done by an outsider? In Menckel (1993), some examples are given of the parts of OHS that can be evaluated by providers and those that should be evaluated by outside experts. Questions like 'Do workers use ear protectors recommended by OHS personnel?' and 'Does the customer follow the rehabilitation programme?' can be evaluated in-house. But outside experts are needed to evaluate questions such as 'Does exposure to noise cause hearing loss?' and 'Is this chair good for a worker with back problems?'

Evaluation of OHS can be performed before a programme is started or implemented (**diagnostic evaluation**), but it is more usual for an experiment to be conducted with one or several different models and reference groups (see Chapters 6 and 7 for further details). This is a before–after evaluation research design (**summative evaluation**). Naturally, evaluation of an ongoing programme can only be performed during or after the programme itself (**formative evaluation**).

All three types of evaluation may have one of two different functions (see Table 2.1). The function of summative evaluation is to control and assess an OHS programme from an outside standpoint. By contrast, the function of formative evaluation is to discuss OHS and change its activities from an inside perspective. In formative evaluation, the evaluator is from the OHS unit to be evaluated (internal evaluation); in summative evaluation, the evaluator comes from outside (external evaluation).

Previously, evaluation was regarded as something designed to be undertaken by experts following the directives of an organization's management (see Table 2.2). Now, it is perceived as a natural part of a

Table 2.1 *Key questions and their relation to summative and formative evaluation*

Questions	Summative evaluation	Formative evaluation
Why and how to be used?	To gain knowledge for assessing operations/individual activities	To gain knowledge for changing operations/individual activities
For whom?	Owner, board, management, clients (personnel)	Management (clients), personnel
By whom?	Outside expert	Member of in-house staff
What?	Goal-result/effect	Operative work
When?	Usually after	Contemporaneously
How often?	Relatively seldom/specific occasions	More frequently/several occasions
How designed?	Quantitative description, statistical compilation	Qualitative description, problem identification, change analysis

Source: Menckel, 1993

Table 2.2 *Changes in evaluation perspectives*

Evaluation 'before'	Evaluation 'now'
Imposed from above	Regarded as an aid
Is a duty or task	Functions as a tool
Takes time away from 'real work'	Perceived as important, worth time
Not integrated in the organization	The organization learns
Highlights only negative results	Shows how we get better
Is complex and requires experts	Is everyone's concern
Is expensive	Should be part of regular work
Quantity over quality	Quantity and quality both important

Source: Adapted from Menckel, 1993

process, a tool that can be employed by everyone in everyday working life for the promotion of change and improvement.

Evaluation therefore has become a way of following up the results of previous processes and obtaining improved knowledge for future operations. In recent years also, there has been a movement in evaluation practice away from the employment of just a single technique to the utilization of a wide range of methods (Weiss, 1972). Choice of method will principally depend on the purpose of the evaluation in question. Previously, evaluation was regarded as 'value-free', while now there is a more pluralistic perspective that encompasses a variety of goals and stakeholders.

Three aspects of OHS evaluation

Donabedian (1988) distinguished three aspects of health care systems – structure (input), process and outcome. Structural or input aspects can be divided into system characteristics (administrative, organizational, physical and financial facilities), provider characteristics (knowledge, specialty training, beliefs/attitudes), and 'patient or client characteristics' (age, gender, health habits, preferences, expectations) (see Hulshof *et al.*, 1998).

Process refers to the actual content of provided care in its technical aspects (activities, continuity of care, etc.). Outcome denotes the effects of care delivered on the health status of patients or populations. Holland (1983) classifies the outcomes of health care according to 'the five Ds' – death, disease, disability, discomfort and dissatisfaction. Other outcome parameters of more proximate relevance in the OHS arena are improved (good) work conditions, functional status, general well-being, satisfaction with care, and return to work.

Process evaluation is the evaluation of health care provided. Two basic questions addressed by process evaluation are: 'Does an intervention reach its target group?' and 'Was the intervention carried out in the way it was planned?' The value of process evaluation should not be underestimated (Hulshof et al., 1998). For new health programmes, knowledge of how (un)successful an outcome was obtained will have the greatest impact on future decision-making. Especially when outcome findings are negative, a thorough process evaluation can provide information on the reason for the negative outcome. Is it lack of implementation? Or, is it a lack of efficiency or effectiveness in the service or programme?

Because a poor outcome does not occur every time there is an error in the provision of care, process data may sometimes be a more sensitive measure of quality than outcome data. Accordingly, in comprehensive evaluation studies, true or quasi-experimental designs for outcome measurements should be combined with process evaluation to monitor how an outcome was achieved.

The systems model in OHS evaluation

The systems model is a frequently used framework for evaluation in HSR. In the risk-oriented preventive occupational health arena, the main goal of OHS is to eliminate or minimize hazards so as to further workers' health (the protection and prevention principle). The outcome of OHS should be tangible in terms of occupational health hazards. Figure 2.1 shows the elements of the OHS system, their more detailed components and their inter-relationships.

According to Kalimo (1986), input into the OHS system – as represented by its resources – includes money, manpower, facilities and technology made available for service provision. Input is transformed into output through the process of the system. Output can be divided into supply and demand, the former referring to the amount, type and quality of the services, the latter to realized demand from the workplaces and their workers. Following Donabedian, a distinction between output and effect is also made by Draaisma (1991) – output being advice from OHS professionals, and effect or outcome being results in terms of better employees' health or diminished health hazards.

Understanding relationships between elements in each OHS subsystem is essential to analysis and evaluation of the system's aspects. Figure 2.1 shows how system concepts can be understood on the basis of the system's elements.

The systems concepts given on the right-hand side of Figure 2.1 refer

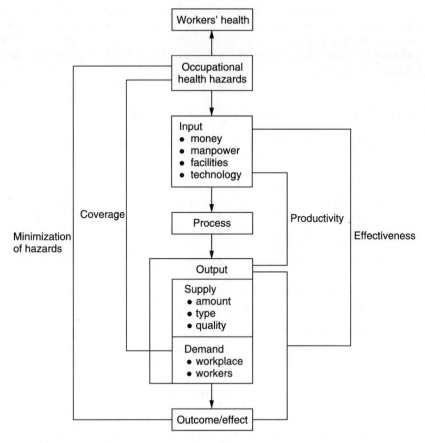

Figure 2.1 *Occupational health hazards, elements of occupational health services and their interrelationships*

to technical aspects. The relationship between output and input is called productivity. Outcome and effect are related to output through effectiveness, and effectiveness is related to input through efficiency, which is often the most important technical systems concept. The systems concepts given on the left-hand side of Figure 2.1 refer to aspects showing the relationships of various system elements to the essential systems objective, namely the prevention of occupational health hazards. Demand is related to occupational health hazards through coverage, which is understood here to refer to OHS that are actually used (i.e. not to services that are available but not used). Finally, there is the most important systems concept, which is the relationship between system outcome and occupational health hazards. This is called the 'minimization of hazards', on the ground that this relationship reflects the results of the occupational health system in terms of its main programme objective.

The systems model provides a good way of reducing an OHS programme or intervention to its basic elements. But it is important to note that we have to measure both process and output to understand why an intervention has been (un)successful. And often it is more feasible to perform only a process evaluation. It can be more sensitive than an outcome evaluation, and its results will be available within a much shorter time period.

Applying the systems model to OHS evaluation

The essential task in empirical studies of OHS is to define system objectives and their subsequent indicators (which are the operational definitions used for statistical analysis).

In Finland, we used the conceptual framework described in Figure 2.1 when developing our national OHS system for farmers. Experiments were conducted using several models and reference groups, and evaluated by means of a before–during–after design. The same model can be used in developing an OHS system for other occupational groups in other settings, or it can be modified for the evaluation of existing OHS systems.

The ultimate goal of the Farmers' OHS (FOHS) experiment in Finland was to lower the incidence and prevalence of work-related diseases among agricultural workers. It was hoped that the overall goal could be achieved through the attainment of a number of intermediate objectives. OHS were to improve farmers' knowledge of health hazards in their work, to change their attitudes and to encourage them to improve their work conditions.

It was realized that a precondition for effective OHS activities was that OHS staff could identify health hazards in farmers' work. In health examinations, nurses and doctors should also be able to identify illness in agricultural workers and those at risk of work-related disease. This process (quantity and quality of health examinations, and identification of occupational health hazards) was subjected to evaluation. Following this step, it was assumed that OHS would provide farmers with sound and easily comprehensible counselling and instructions (= output), which would then help to improve their work conditions and persuade them to use personal protective equipment.

The FOHS experiment did not clearly indicate when the desired effects were assumed to materialize. In the evaluators' view, effects on work-related morbidity could not be expected for many years, but there was the possibility of immediate effects in terms of increased use of personal protectors and improvements in work conditions. In general, it is good to have indicators or measures that can be used in a shorter time span rather than waiting for the ultimate goal of a programme or intervention to be realized. Nevertheless, these intermediate objectives have to be such that there are good grounds for believing them to be directly related to outcome objectives.

Figure 2.2 has the same OHS conceptual model elements as Figure 2.1. But the various (outcome/effect) objectives, the means for achieving them, and the relationship between OHS and other primary health care activities are described in greater detail. Figure 2.2 shows the various

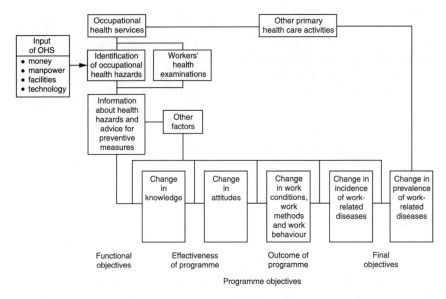

Figure 2.2 *A detailed model of the objectives of occupational health service experiments and their evaluation*

means available for influencing occupational health hazards and, thereby, the incidence and prevalence of work-related diseases. These are what we call 'functional objectives'. An OHS programme can be evaluated at any level of its objectives, but the preceding objectives in the hierarchy must also be included at the level chosen. This highlights the importance of combining process evaluation with outcome evaluation. Without such a combination, one cannot tell whether the success or failure of a programme is due to theory or process.

One important issue remains to be discussed. In what does the outcome/effect of an OHS intervention consist? Might it not be, for example, that the noise level in a factory has fallen to a safe level (under 85 dB) and that workers no longer need to use ear protectors? Of course, if this happens, the ultimate goal of OHS will be realized – there will be no new cases of hearing loss. But can such an outcome/effect be attained solely through OHS activity? Or are there other actors who have an impact on the desired outcome? Do we still need decision-making and money from the employer? And perhaps also some input on the part of the workers?

Look at Figure 2.2 and consider the possibility that OHS personnel have taken all the right steps – identified the health hazard (i.e. the noise) correctly, provided good factual information about the hazard, and stressed the importance of eliminating it to both employer and employees. Perhaps, changes in their knowledge and attitudes have taken place. But, for some reason, the employer may have decided not to eliminate the noise sufficiently, or perhaps company engineers are incapable of doing it. Is this a failure on the part of OHS? Maybe not. They succeeded in all steps of the process that could be controlled in some degree only by them. But they did not attain the final goal of cutting down the noise level to under 85 dB.

At least in this example, let us think about the fact that the goals of OHS are not that simple to define, and the outcomes have many dimensions. There are also many other actors involved in the decisions needed to eliminate occupational health hazards in real workplaces. When planning the evaluation of an OHS system, however, it is always possible to establish criteria and measurable indicators of outcomes. These criteria may vary according to the OHS system and the purpose of the evaluation research.

Conclusions

The evaluation of OHS is not an easy task. We can do it in many ways, and from many points of view, for instance from the viewpoints of society, the clients and service providers. It may help us, the providers of services, to have trust in our own work, which is often difficult in prevention without evaluation. The Farmers' Occupational Health Services (FOHS) experiment, with its quasi-experimental design, is a unique example of a successful, national-level evaluation study, which has been nationally implemented and is still (1998) continually evaluated and developed. And in the FOHS experiment these same principles and the systems model have been applied. In these days of limited resources and too great a belief in the market economy, it is of utmost importance to demonstrate to the financers of occupational health services that we can effectively achieve the ultimate goal of OHS, which is to decrease the incidence and prevalence of work-related diseases and to enhance the working ability of the working population.

References and further reading

Black, N. (1996) Why we need observational studies to evaluate the effectiveness of health care. *Br. Med. J.*, **312**, 1215-18.

Campbell, D.T. and Stanley, J.C. (1963) Experimental and quasi-experimental designs for research. Reprinted from *Handbook of Research on Teaching*. Boston, MA: Houghton Mifflin.

van Dijk, F.J.H., de Kort, W. and Verbeek, J.H.A.M. (1993) Quality assessment of occupational health care instruments. *Occup. Med.*, **43** (Suppl. 1), 28-33.

Donabedian, A. (1988) The quality of care. How can it be assessed? *JAMA*, **260**, 1743-8.

Draaisma, D. (1991) A conceptual approach for the evaluation of the quality and effectiveness of occupational health care. In: *New Trends and Developments in Occupational Health Services* (Rantanen, J. and Lehtinen, S., eds), International Congress Series 890. Amsterdam: Excerpta Medica, pp. 49-54.

Guidotti, T.L., Cowell, J.W.F., Jamieson, G.G. and Engelberg, A.L. (1989) Program evaluation. In: *Occupational Health Services, a Practical Approach*. Chicago: AMA.

Holland, W.W. (ed.) (1983) *Evaluation of Health Care*. Oxford: Oxford University Press.

Hulshof, C.T.J., Verbeek, J.H.A.M. and van Dijk, F.J.H. (1993) Development and evaluation of an occupational health services programme on the prevention and control of effects of vibration. *Occup. Med.*, **43** (Suppl 1), 38-42.

Hulshof, C.T.J., Verbeek, J.H.A.M., van Dijk, F.J.H., van der Weide, W.E. and Braam, I.T.J. (1998) Evaluation research in Occupational Health Services. General principles and a model for OHS evaluation. In: *Prevention and Control of Adverse Effects of Whole-body Vibration. An Evaluation Study in Occupational Health Services* (Hulshof, C.T.J., ed.). Wageningen: University of Amsterdam/Drukkerij Ponsen amp Looijen bv.

Husman, K. (1993) Principles and pitfalls in health services research in occupational health systems. *Occup. Med.*, **43** (Suppl 1), 10-14.

Husman, K., Notkola, V., Virolainen, R., Tupi, K., Nuutinen, J., Penttinen, J. and Heikkonen, J. (1988) Farmers' occupational health program in Finland, 1979–1988. *Scand. J. Work Environ. Hlth*, **14** (Suppl 1), 118-20.

Husman, K. and Notkola, V. (1991) Theory, research and practice in the planning, implementation and evaluation of occupational health services. In: *New Trends and Developments in Occupational Health Services* (Rantanen, J and Lehtinen, S., eds), International Congress Series 890. Amsterdam: Excerpta Medica, pp. 39-47.

International Labour Office (ILO) (1985) *Occupational Health Services Convention 1985*. Geneva: ILO, Convention No. 161.

Kalimo, E. (1986) Methodological issues of health systems research in the evaluation of occupational health services. In: *Occupational Health as a Component of Primary Health Care*. Proceedings of a WHO Meeting 9–13 September 1985, Turku, Finland (J. Järvisalo, E. Kalimo, M. Lamberg and J. Rantanen, eds). Publications of the National Board of Health, Finland, pp. 27–36.

Macdonal, E.B. (ed.), Agius, R.M., McCloy, E.C., McCulloch, W.J.M., Miller, D.M., Paterson, J.C. and Whitaker, S. (1995) *Quality and Audit in Occupational Health*. London: Faculty of Occupational Medicine of the Royal College of Physicians of London.

Menckel, E. (1993) *Evaluating and Promoting change in Occupational Health Services – Models and Applications*. Stockholm: The Swedish Work Environment Fund.

Plomp, H.N. (1993) Workers' attitudes toward the occupational physician. *J. Occup. Med.*, **34**, 9.

Pransky, G. and Himmelstein, J. (1996) Outcomes research: implications for occupational health. *Am. J. Ind. Med.*, **29**, 573-83.

Räsänen, K., Notkola, V., Kankaanpää, E., Peurala, M. and Husman, K. (1993) Role of the occupational health services as a part of illness-related primary care in Finland. *Occup. Med.*, **43** (Suppl 1), 23-7.

Räsänen, K. (1998) *Illness-related Care Within Occupational Health Services. Relationship with General Primary Care, Work-related Illness and Workplace Health Promotion in Finland*. Kuopio University Publications D. Medical Sciences 142. Kuopio, Finland.

Rossi, P.H. and Freeman, H.E. (1989) *Evaluation. A Systematic Approach*, 4th edn. Beverly Hills, CA: Sage Publications.

Schulte, P.A., Goldenhar, L.M. and Connally, L.B. (1996) Intervention research: science, skills, and strategies. *Am. J. Ind. Med.*, **29**, 285-8.

Shortell, S.M. and Richardson, W.C. (1989) *Health Program Evaluation*, 4th edn. Beverly Hills, CA: Sage Publications.

Suchman, E.A. (1967) *Evaluative Research. Principles and Practice in Public Service and Social Action Program*. New York: Russell Sage Foundation.

Wannag, A. and Nord, E. (1993) Work content of Norwegian occupational physicians. *Scand. J. Work Environ. Hlth*, **19**, 394-8.

Weiss, C.H (1972) *Evaluation Research. Methods for Assessing Program Effectiveness*. (Methods of Social Science Series). Englewood Cliffs, NJ: Prentice-Hall.

WHO (1982) *Evaluation of Occupational Health and Industrial Hygiene Services*. Report on a WHO Working Group. Copenhagen: WHO Euro Reports and Studies 56.

WHO (1984) *Glossary of Terms Used in the 'Health for All' series No. 1–8.* ('Health for All' Series No 9). Geneva: WHO.

WHO (1985) *Identification and Control of Work-related diseases*. Geneva: WHO Technical Report Series 714.

WHO (1990) Occupational health services. An overview. *Regional Publications European Series No 26*. Geneva: WHO.

3

Evaluation, quality assurance, quality improvement and research

Jos Verbeek, Carel Hulshof and Willeke van der Weide

For strategic and substantive reasons, quality of care should receive greater attention in occupational health. Although most governments guarantee some minimum standard of quality, much can still be gained from quality improvement. It is best to concentrate on the process rather than the outcome of care, since this is more likely to reflect the quality of occupational health services. Instruments include the development of guidelines, scientific-evaluation research, literature databases like Medline, and satisfaction surveys among patients and employers. Much depends on the willingness of quality-improvement teams to devote time and energy to problems signalled by dissatisfied stakeholders. This chapter emphasizes the importance of utilization of research literature by OHS professionals and key points are illustrated by means of the story of an occupational physician.

Problems with the quality of occupational health services (OHS) are more and more troublesome in a market-oriented occupational health setting. Accordingly, there is a great need for assessment of quality. This can best be based on a systems model of occupational health, which stresses the need for careful examination of opportunities to improve services. Different stakeholders, such as the government, health-care professionals and scientists, all have their own contribution to make. The government should set minimum standards for quality in occupational health. Evidence of effectiveness is the basis for guidelines laid down by professionals. These guidelines can then be audited in medical practice, which should lead to quality improvement.

The occupational physician meets the concept of quality

An occupational physician returns from a meeting with the manager of a company that buys services from his OHS unit. He is frustrated. He is working hard, doing the best he can. He has used all his professional abilities to increase the health of workers at a particular company. Rather than gratitude, he has received a great deal of criticism. Management thinks the absenteeism rate is too high. Workers are not satisfied with the back school that the occupational physician has organized. 'The services you provide do not solve my problems', is what the manager has told him. These words are still ringing in his ears. Back at his service unit, his own supervisor is not pleased to have a dissatisfied customer. To solve the problem, he proposes that the occupational physician no longer provides services to this company, and swaps work with his colleague. He hesitates, but accepts the offer. It frees him from a pain in the neck.

This might be an example from everyday life that you recognize. But the solution to the problem of a dissatisfied customer does not seem very efficient. What has evaluation, quality assurance and research got to offer in preventing such 'pains in the neck'?

Quality assurance has long been recognized as a method to improve the quality of products in industry – so much so that modern management does not seem to be possible without reference to quality assurance. But many want to go beyond the concept of assurance and talk about quality improvement. Some use the term 'Total Quality Management' (TQM) for the strategy by which all aspects of company and production processes are continuously improved.

Occupational health care can be seen as a part of this Total Quality Management (Berwick, 1990). Accordingly, it is important to have some idea of the quality of occupational health care. In this chapter, we will first go through some important notions about quality of care, and try to find out if there is a quality problem. Then, we will examine possible solutions to quality problems that can be provided by the medical profession, society, and the scientific community.

Do OHS have a quality problem?

Quality is defined by the International Standards Organization (ISO) as 'the totality of features and characteristics of a product or service that bear on its ability to satisfy stated or implied needs' (ISO, 1991). We find this a useful definition, which can also be applied to OHS. But even though the statement appears robust, many questions can be asked about it. For example, whose needs have to be satisfied? It is quite possible that different users have different needs. This means that there is no such thing as quality *per se*, but that the concept of quality should always be referred to from the point of view of a potential user of a product or service.

It is easy to see that such a concept of quality overlaps with the idea of evaluation. In evaluation, one tries to assess the capacity of a programme to achieve certain aims or goals. And, also in evaluation, it is important to make clear whom you are working for. See also Chapters 2 (Husman) and 4 (Øvretveit).

Context and special features of OHS

Especially in occupational health, we have to deal with the problem of different service users. Employers and employees, in particular, usually have different needs in relation to occupational health care. Draaisma and colleagues (1991) carried out a questionnaire survey of employers, employees and OHS staff with regard to their opinions on the quality of occupational health care in The Netherlands. Responses showed that both employers and employees thought that OHS should pay greater attention to work conditions and occupational rehabilitation. Employees confided less in OHS organizations that solely provided occupational rehabilitation. However, workers' councils and management differed in their opinions of the effectiveness of OHS in eliminating health hazards.

Further, to be able to speak about quality in occupational health, we need an idea about how it is functioning and what its aims are. In this context, it is good to use a systems model of health care, as first described by Donabedian and later adapted by Husman for the occupational health arena (Donabedian, 1988).

Figure 3.1 shows the most important elements in a model for occupational health. The arrow at the bottom represents the causal processes that lead to occupational diseases, work-related disorders, or occupational disabilities. It is the main goal of OHS to prevent these problems, either by intervening in the causal process or by eliminating their causes directly. This is clarified in the figure by using italics to demonstrate an example of noise and hearing problems. A decrease in the incidence and

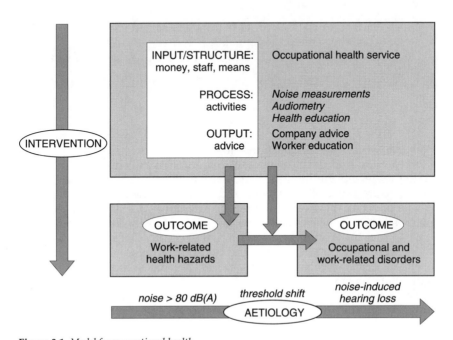

Figure 3.1 *Model for occupational health*

prevalence of such problems is usually called the **outcome** of an occupational health intervention. Figures on such health outcomes can be used to measure the quality of OHS (Pransky and Himmelstein, 1996). The greater their ability to improve the outcome, the better is its quality. But, before conclusions are drawn solely on the basis of outcome, we should take a look at the service *process* .

The vertical arrows in the figure represent different aspects of the interventions that make up the core of occupational health. Jointly, we call them the **process** of occupational health intervention. Here, it is also useful to look at **input** in terms of finances, professional resources and instruments – i.e. the **structure** that makes it possible to carry out the process. And processes usually generate some form of **output**, such as concrete advice to a company or worker.

Since implementation of the output is often beyond the power of the occupational physician, it is important to take the process of occupational health intervention into consideration when looking at the quality obtained. In other medical specialties, such as nursing, psychotherapy and rehabilitation medicine, there are also many factors beyond the scope of the professional that may generate a particular health outcome. In the case of these specialties, more can be learned about quality by examining process of care rather than its outcome. Further, some authors have argued that process data are more sensitive and informative measures of quality than outcome data in health care (Davies and Crombie, 1995). On this line of thinking, variation in professional practice is often regarded as an indicator of low quality.

This systems model of occupational health makes it possible to ask questions about its quality:

- Do all OHS organizations provide the same services?
- Do they use the same professionals?
- Does the output of OHS vary between professionals or types of service units?

State of current knowledge

Some answers to the questions above can be given by the scientific literature. To find out how well OHS are doing, Hulshof and colleagues (1998) reviewed the literature on evaluation and quality in the occupational health arena. They categorized studies on the basis of the systems model of occupational health described in Figure 3.1. Although there are many studies of the efficacy of certain types of interventions, they found only 48 that dealt with the evaluation of everyday OHS practice. Most of these were aimed at evaluating the input or structure of services. However, 13 dealt with aspects of process, six measured output, and 11 looked at outcome.

The methodological quality of most studies was found to be rather low. The studies of input or structure were almost all of a descriptive nature, and did not use a design that would make it possible to draw conclusions about the effectiveness of the services provided. It turned out that occupational health consultation and occupational rehabilitation were scarcely studied at all, which contrasts with the large amount of time spent on these topics by occupational physicians.

Of the five studies concerned with the process of pre-employment examinations, only one was positive about quality – one that dealt with the very specific situation of occupational asthma among bakers. For output and outcome of pre-employment examinations, one single, negative study was found. Wide variation in the practice of pre-employment examinations was demonstrated by de Kort (1992). He used data on 130 job applicants judged as medically fit for the tasks in question, and 45 applicants judged as unfit. A panel of five experienced occupational physicians reassessed these data. In 20% of all cases their opinion was opposite to that of the original physician. In only 64% of cases did the panel agree with the original physician. Hulshof and colleagues conclude that pre-employment examinations lack effectiveness and efficiency, and advise that the instrument should no longer be used as a means of personnel selection. As a proviso, they add that it might have a place in certain very specific situations.

By contrast, the quality of the process of periodic health surveillance and workplace surveys was found to be good, although they did not automatically guarantee a good outcome in health terms. Hulshof and colleagues take the view that there should be much more effort directed at evaluation studies, and also at improvement of the methodological quality of these studies.

Another way of obtaining data on the quality of OHS is to utilize administrative systems of the kind advocated by the Agency for Health Care Policy and Research (AHCPR, 1995). For example, in The Netherlands, the Health and Safety Office for the Construction Industry (Arbouw) administers all the activities of occupational physicians in that industry. Since reimbursement of these activities is based on the system, we can attribute at least some validity to these data.

Figure 3.2 shows the percentage of workers diagnosed with noise-induced hearing loss for 40 OHS units and 63 000 occupational health consultations. It can be seen that this percentage ranges from 0 to 17.5. As this large body of data all concerns construction workers under more or less the same work conditions, the proportion of workers with hearing loss should be about the same across OHS units. But the variation in diagnoses is large, and – accordingly – quality in diagnosing noise-induced hearing loss cannot be expected to be high.

A third indication that OHS might have a quality problem is the change in orientation from being a more-or-less public institution towards a profit-making business in a competitive market. For example, in both The Netherlands and Sweden, OHS have been privatized and become increasingly market-oriented in recent years. Employers have to pay for OHS, and are wondering where the benefits lie. The same question is being asked by governments. If we take occupational health seriously as an essential part of public health, there should be some guarantee of a minimum acceptable level of OHS quality. It is up to the government to set such a standard.

We conclude that questions of quality and effectiveness can no longer

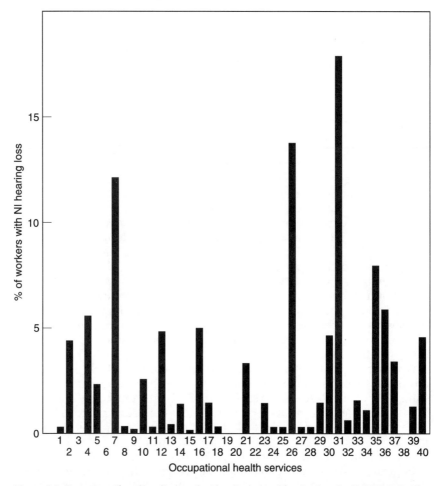

Figure 3.2 *Percentage of workers diagnosed with noise-induced hearing loss for 40 OHS units: the variation in diagnoses is large*

be avoided. Quality problems in OHS probably occur frequently. And they are evident at different levels – at company level, at a professional and scientific level, and at a governmental level.

Solutions to quality problems

Solutions to quality problems can be found at the level at which they arise. This means that all the stakeholders involved have to play their own role – occupational physicians as a professional group, OHS as an organization, scientists in the field of occupational health, and the government.

Government-sponsored quality assurance in The Netherlands

Occupational health is an essential public-health function, which should not be left to open-market competition. At least from the point of view of workers' health, minimum quality standards for OHS should be guaranteed by government measures. But even from a commercial point of view, OHS can benefit from the kinds of basic standards demonstrated by the ISO-9000 series on quality management. Such standards are intended to provide purchaser satisfaction, and offer confidence in suppliers' quality systems (ISO, 1991).

In The Netherlands, the government has opted for a certification procedure to guarantee a minimum standard of quality. Every employer in The Netherlands is obliged to hire a certified OHS organization to provide at least the following four services:

- risk identification and evaluation;
- regular health examinations;
- occupational rehabilitation;
- occupational health consultations.

In the future, it is intended that the certification process will be carried out by an independent body. At the moment, it is performed by the Ministry of Social Affairs. The process consists of three phases, and is carried out every four years.

The structure of OHS should guarantee a sufficient level of professionalism. At least four professionals should be part of the staff of any OHS organization:

- occupational physician;
- occupational hygienist;
- safety engineer;
- organization specialist.

Each OHS unit should have a quality assurance system based on ISO-9001, which implies that all procedures are written down in a quality handbook. This is the typical industrial way of conducting quality assurance in a strict sense. But, at a third phase, the certifying body checks whether the services provided to companies are of sufficient quality.

Unfortunately, only the last part is really content-related, and – even so – it is still not very well developed. No content-related guidelines or criteria exist, against which the quality of services provided can be measured. The only check is whether the services comply with the law.

Returning to our harassed physician in the example above, we might wonder if a better certification procedure could have prevented his predicament. But since the certification procedure is so weakly content-related, we doubt that this is a solution.

Quality assurance by the medical profession

Guideline development

A worker with low-back pain was referred by his supervisor to our occupational physician. He is a packer in an industrial enterprise, but is unable to carry out his job tasks because of back pain. Our physician sends him to a back school organized by his OHS physiotherapist. After three months, the patient is still not back at work, and he still experiences back pain. His supervisor is not pleased, the worker is not content, and the physician feels as if he is doing everything wrong. He wonders if there is a right way of going about things.

It is one of the typical features of being a professional that society trusts the profession to which the person belongs. This applies especially in medicine, and doctors are imbued with a special kind of 'quality'. This highlights the role occupational physicians have to play in quality assurance.

One way to eliminate unacceptable variations in practice is to develop guidelines. Professional guidelines are complementary to the quality-certification process. But the process is usually directed at business processes separate from content. The ISO-9000 quality standard assures that what companies state they are doing is really done – but without saying anything about the product or service itself. Guidelines can help fill this gap.

In the context we are considering, according to Grimshaw and Russell (1993), guidelines are systematically developed statements designed to assist practitioner decisions about appropriate health care for specific clinical circumstances. van der Weide and colleagues (1998a) have described a method to develop and evaluate guidelines for occupational physicians. They argue, in line with many other authors (Grol, 1993; Davies and Crombie, 1995), that guidelines should be formed on the basis of scientific evidence. But, since it is impossible to get scientific evidence to bear on every aspect of clinical practice, additional methods are needed. Consensus among experts is a popular route to take in this context. Guidelines are usually provided by a specialist organization specifically for its members. In the USA, for example, the American College of Occupational and Environmental Medicine has published a set of guidelines for occupational physicians (ACOEM, 1997). And, in The Netherlands, the Dutch Association of Occupational Physicians is working on guidelines for the rehabilitation of workers with low-back pain and those with mental problems.

Sometimes, governmental organizations are also involved. For example, the American Agency for Health Care Policy and Research has published guidelines on many clinical topics, including low-back pain (Bigos et al., 1994). Some of these are available on the internet at http://text.nlm.nih.gov/

An example of a guideline to occupational physicians for the rehabilitation of workers with low-back pain is given by van der Weide and colleagues (1997b, 1998b). This guideline might be of help to our occupational physician. The aim of the guideline is to assist physicians in making decisions in the return-to-work process. The authors hope that occupational physicians can prevent unnecessary absence from work and unnecessary long-term disability. They base their guideline on a systematic review of studies of the efficacy of conventional treatment for low-back pain (van der Weide, 1997a). From the guideline, it can be concluded that there is no place for back schools in the treatment or rehabilitation of workers with low-back pain – even though this is not stated explicitly.

zn the absence of guidelines, Sackett and colleagues (1997) recommend that occupational professionals perform their own literature survey. Everyone with access to the internet can freely search the medical literature, as abstracted in Medline at http://www.ncbi.nlm.gov/PubMed. If our occupational physician had done so he would, for example, have found the study of Daltroy and colleagues (1997), who found no evidence of an effect of attending back school on sickness absence or on return to work in a randomized 5-year follow-up study. This might have made him wary of the possible effects of back schools.

Guidelines are not only of use for the individual practitioner. When implemented on a large scale, they can substantially improve the quality of medical care. See, for example, the review by Grimshaw and Russell (1993). However, there are many factors that influence the implementation of guidelines, such as the involvement of practitioners in development and try-out (Wensing and Grol, 1994). Accordingly, if guidelines are used to improve quality of care, adequate attention should be paid to the implementation phase.

Evaluation of daily practice and medical audit

Having discovered guidelines for rehabilitation of patients with low-back pain, our occupational physician wants to find out if he is doing all right with all his patients. In collaboration with a colleague, he embarks upon an audit of patient charts.

Practice guidelines describe a standard way of carrying out professional activities. They enable us to test practice against certain standards. This is more or less similar to the process of medical audit, which is widespread in the UK (and discussed in greater detail elsewhere in this book).

A formal definition of medical audit is that it is the systematic, critical analysis of the quality of medical care, including the procedures used for diagnosis and treatment, the use of resources, and the resulting outcome and quality of life for the patient (Faculty of Occupational Medicine, 1995). Agius (1990) has reported extensively on the results of this type of medical audit. (See also Chapter 5 by Agius *et al.* in this book.)

In our view, however, the process of medical audit can be substantially improved by the utilization of explicit guidelines. Further, such guidelines can and should be translated into performance indicators and quality criteria. An indicator of performance can be defined as an essential element in care that gives a valid and representative picture of its quality. Indicators can be selected for aspects of structure, process or outcome, according to what is in focus.

Quality indicators are also called performance measures by some authors. Indicators should be made operational by criteria, or what are called review criteria. A criterion gives an answer to the question of what is appropriate or desirable. To be able to take patient characteristics into account, these criteria should be formulated in 'if–then' statements. If a patient has a certain characteristic, then the physician should perform a specific action. How such explicit criteria should be used is self-evident. They are objective, can be used by external assessors, and have high reliability.

In the example of low-back pain and return to work an important indicator of performance or quality is encouragement of physical activity. *If* a patient has a diagnosis of non-specific low-back pain, *then* advice to stay active or return to work should be given. Accordingly, the criterion of good care is that such advice is given. If it is given, the quality of care is good; if it is not, quality is insufficient. This instrument for quality assessment is elaborated in greater detail by van der Weide and colleagues (1998a), and by the AHCPR (1995).

> Our occupational physician and his colleague constructed some simple performance measures for back pain diagnosis and psychosocial problems. Using these indicators, they reviewed 50 patient charts. They found that they did not have a proper diagnosis in 50% of cases, and that – if psychosocial problems were present in 40% of these – proper advice or treatment was lacking. They decided to start an improvement project to investigate low-back pain diagnoses and interventions for psychosocial problems.

The role and contribution of research

What is the role of research in quality improvement? Is it just a matter of improving procedures and trying to improve the performance of the individual practitioner? Or do we need help from the scientific community? Of course, the answer to the latter question is 'Yes'. Science has a major role to play, as can be concluded not least from the need to have guidelines with a scientific foundation.

Berwick (1990) argues that the question of the quality of health care can be divided into four important components:

- Is the purpose of care clear?
- Is practice efficacious?
- Are clinical decisions appropriate?
- Is care provided according to guidelines?

From consideration of these sub-questions, it emerges that there are roles for policymakers, scientists and managers to perform alongside professionals working in the field.

To improve quality of care, we need to know which interventions or treatments are working and which are not. Usually, many articles can be found on a specific topic, but it is rather difficult to find evidence and draw conclusions with regard to efficacy. Sackett and colleagues (1997) argue that all medical professionals themselves should be able to find the best solution to a clinical problem from evidence in the literature. They have constructed a list of central clinical tasks that can be approached in a similar manner, such as diagnosis, aetiology, prognosis, therapy and prevention. They provide detailed guidelines concerning how to extract the best evidence from the literature on these topics.

Fortunately, much of this work has been done by others in the form of systematic literature reviews. One of the main tasks of the Cochrane Collaboration has been to prepare and maintain systematic reviews, with the voluntary assistance of scientists all over the world (Oxman, 1994). The results of these systematic reviews are available on quarterly distributed CD-ROMs (The Cochrane Library, ISBN 1-901868-05-2, BMJ, London).

Excellent reviews can be found on topics such as treatment of back pain, smoking cessation, and hepatitis-B vaccination. One of the main advantages of systematic over narrative review lies in the manner in which the literature is searched, the information abstracted and evidence built up. Some authors give the name meta-analysis to this procedure (Petitti, 1994), but meta-analysis is usually distinguished from systematic review. In a meta-analysis, it is possible statistically to pool the results of many studies into one outcome parameter, e.g. a pooled odds ratio. Due to the heterogeneity of outcome parameters or interventions, such statistical pooling is not usually possible in the case of systematic reviews.

Despite the interest in studying health outcomes, researchers have only recently turned their attention to the concerns of working populations and the impact of medical care on vocational status (Pransky and Himmelstein, 1996). Apart from health outcomes, one of the main vocational outcome parameters in occupational health is sickness absence. Accordingly, systematic reviews should also be directed at this type of outcome measure.

A good example of a systematic review is the one conducted by van der Weide and colleagues (1997a) on the vocational outcome of interventions for low-back pain. By contrast with other reviews of musculoskeletal problems, the researchers selected only studies with a vocational outcome – on the grounds that this is the outcome of primary interest for the occupational physician. Most of the studies found defined outcome in terms of the percentage of workers returning to work or the mean number of days of sickness absence.

The studies were then assigned a value for methodological quality, which was used to weigh each study's contribution to the final evidence. Unfortunately, the researchers found only very few studies that were of high methodological quality.

A further drawback of most of the studies was an insufficient number of participants. Sickness absence and return to work are influenced by many factors, and show high variance. This means that a large study group is usually required to draw significant conclusions where there is a negative outcome.

For negative studies, van der Weide and colleagues calculated in 1997 the number of participants needed to detect a 25% difference between treatment and reference groups with a = 0.05 and 80% power. If calculated sample size was above actual sample size, the power of the study was rated as sufficient to warrant a true negative result. The final results of their literature review were rated by so-called levels of evidence, according to methodological quality and the number of studies with positive and negative outcomes (Bigos et al., 1994).

The conclusions of the review are shown in Table 3.1. It is shown that there is only moderate to limited evidence for the efficacy of interventions. For practice guidelines, they advocate that bed rest should be limited or even avoided, and that normal activity should be continued as much as possible. If only conventional treatment for patients with acute low-back pain is considered, then spinal manipulation is the best option. In cases of chronic low-back pain, anti-depressants can be helpful. They also advocate exercise and education programmes in an occupational setting, although there was not enough positive evidence to conclude that such interventions are effective. In sum, the role of research in this context is to contribute to the amount of evidence on the effectiveness of an intervention to reduce a specific unfavourable health outcome.

Importance of study design

Certain research designs are supposed to contribute more in the way of evidence than others (according to their methodological quality). In clinical research, an experiment or randomized controlled trial (RCT) is regarded as the 'gold standard' because of its high internal validity. This high validity is mainly due to the randomization procedure, which substantially lowers the risk of biased results.

Table 3.1 *Evidence for the efficacy of interventions for acute low-back pain with a vocational outcome*

	Outcome						
	Positive		*Negative*				
Quality	*H*	*L*	*H*	*L*	*H*	*L*	
Power				*Suf.*		*Insuf.*	*Evidence*
NSAIDS							
vs placebo						3	No
vs topical						1	No
Little bed rest							
vs more	1	1	1	1			Moderate
Spinal manip.							
vs placebo	1					2	Limited
vs alternative	1	1				1	Moderate
School/exercise							
vs placebo		1	1				No
vs alternative		1	1		1	2	No
Case management							
vs placebo					1		No
vs alternative		1				2	No
Total	3	5	3	1	2	11	

The RCT has the highest credibility in terms of evidence of effectiveness. In more general terms, it can be described as having a true experimental pre-test–post-test control group design. Individuals or populations are divided into an experimental and a control group through random assignment. The experimental group receives the intervention or prevention programme, and the control group receives a competing intervention. The latter is the alternative against which the experimental intervention is compared (Meinert, 1986). In interventions at an individual level, such as in occupational rehabilitation, this design is to be preferred to others. Good examples of RCTs in occupational health are the studies reported in Malmivaara *et al.* (1995) and van der Weide *et al.* (1998b).

Black (1996), however, has drawn attention to the limitations of the RCT design. He argues that RCTs may sometimes be unnecessary, inappropriate, impossible, or even inadequate. In his view, it is in particular the low *external* validity of many RCTs that is often overlooked. It is stated by Black that RCTs 'generally offer an indication of the efficacy of an intervention rather than its effectiveness in everyday practice'.

For some problems, observational studies are more feasible than RCTs. This holds especially in the case of evaluation research in occupational health care. In particular, when occupational health interventions are directed at groups in order to improve work conditions or to provide education, randomization at an individual level is not possible. This problem may sometimes be solved by randomizing on a population base, such as a number of plants or departments. But a drawback of this approach is that it requires very large sample sizes, which are often difficult to organize and keep under control.

In OHS research therefore, the quasi-experimental study design is often the one adopted. Quasi-experimental designs make use of control groups that are not selected through random assignment but by techniques such as matching or stratification. The results of an intervention are determined over time before and after the implementation of an intervention. This design is classically described by Cook and Campbell (1979). In this context, it involves assigning plants, departments or OHS units to an experimental and a control group. (See also Chapter 4, John Øvretveit.)

A less powerful but widely used design is the one-group pre-test–post-test design, in which the target group acts as its own control. The conclusiveness of findings may then be increased by replication of the study in another population, or by increasing the number of observations before and after the intervention. Such a time-series design ideally includes at least three measurements before, and three after the intervention has taken place. To be valid, changes in trends must be consistent for the different plants or departments, and the same intervention must have been introduced at different times.

A good example of a quasi-experimental study is reported in Hulshof *et al.* (1998). Following a comprehensive study of the effects of whole-body vibration and possible interventions, the researchers decided to evaluate these interventions in practice. Eight OHS organizations were assigned to an experimental group, and six to a control group. The experimental group was trained in performance of the programme, and the control group was asked to provide care as usual. At baseline, there were no differences between the experimental and control groups.

Unfortunately, after the intervention was carried out, no statistically significant or meaningful reduction in the mean whole-body vibration exposure level could be demonstrated. But the researchers also studied the process by which the intervention was designed to have an effect.

A detailed process evaluation revealed improvement in relation to intermediate objectives, such as increased company awareness of whole-body vibration, improved attitude and intended behaviour on the part of forklift drivers, and increased knowledge on the part of professionals and managers. However, the number of control measures for which implementation could be observed was too low. This explained the negative result. It was concluded that a further study, with a larger sample size, a longer follow-up, and greater focus on implementation was necessary. For us, it provides a good example of the usefulness of process evaluation in a research setting.

Role of patient and customer satisfaction

The effectiveness of health care is not only determined by quality parameters, but also by the acceptance of the parties involved. Acceptance is closely associated with patients' or populations' *satisfaction* with care. By some authors, satisfaction is regarded as a process measure – important as a means of gaining acceptance of and participation in the service being provided. By others, patient satisfaction is considered as one of the desired outcomes of care, even an element in health status itself (Donabedian, 1988). Patient or customer satisfaction is regarded as an important indicator of a possible lack of quality, and can be used to improve quality of services. There are only very few studies of the satisfaction of patients or customers with occupational health interventions (Bosma *et al.*, 1996).

Comparing evaluation, research and quality terminology

One of the problems of evaluation research is that terminology differs according to discipline. The terminologies of the various disciplines involved are compared in Table 3.2. Most of the items in the table have been elucidated in the preceding text. 'Run chart' and 'control chart', however, are terms that stem from statistical quality-assurance in industry, and are not widely used in the health-care arena. Nevertheless, they can be practical instruments for measuring deviance from normal procedures or services. For example, waiting times can be measured on a regular basis, and control charts employed to ascertain on which days waiting times were abnormally long in a statistical sense. Possible causes and possibilities for improvement should be looked into with regard to these days (Carey and Lloyd, 1997).

Table 3.2 *Comparability and terminology of study designs in different scientific disciplines*

Rank order	Evaluation study (social sciences)	Clinical research/ observational epidemiology	Quality assurance/ quality improvement
1	True experiment pre-/post test control group design	Randomized controlled trial Community intervention trial	
2	Quasi-experimental design	Cohort study Case control study	
3	Non-experimental design: e.g. time series	Patient series Descriptive study	Run chart/ control chart
4	Judgemental design		Peer review Audit Satisfaction with care
	Process evaluation	Compliance Descriptive study	Audit Certification Guidelines Satisfaction

Quality improvement in OHS – a better solution

Berwick and colleagues (1990) have claimed health care has many short-comings, such as still-rising prices, long waiting periods for service, an allegedly rising error rate and evidence of greed and fraud in some sectors. No doubt, the same shortcomings are to be found in occupational health care, but what is more important is that they are evident in many other industry and service sectors.

According to Berwick and colleagues, only the fittest sectors will survive. They argue that survival is closely linked to responding to customers' needs and to a policy of continuous quality improvement. Accordingly, they heavily stress the need for quality improvement in health care to overcome current shortcomings.

The authors assert that this is not only an issue for doctors, but that many different stakeholders are involved – secretaries, occupational hygienists, managers, and so on. Accordingly, quality improvement involves a team of workers. Basically, every quality improvement project has to follow five steps:

1 Select a problem to work on.
2 Organize a team to carry out the improvement project.
3 Diagnose the problem.
4 Plan, test and implement a remedy.
5 Check and monitor performance.

The start of a quality improvement cycle might be a complaining customer or patient, or a dissatisfied professional. Several different instruments are available for diagnosing the problem, such as flow charts to describe the processes, or fishbone diagrams to use for brainstorming sessions about possible causes of the undesirable outcome.

It is for research to provide the largest possible amount of evidence necessary for improvement in the quality of care. Apart from providing evidence of effectiveness of interventions, research should be directed towards the development of sensitive and specific methods for practitioners to monitor and evaluate performance and quality of care (Carey and Lloyd, 1997). In the end, it is up to the manager of an OHS unit and the professionals working there to ensure that they succeed in providing services to their customers of the highest possible quality.

Our occupational physician was not satisfied with what was happening. He decided to find out what had gone wrong, and how he could prevent things from continuing to go wrong. He persuaded his manager to form a quality improvement team. The first problem addressed by the team was the dissatisfied company manager. The team formulated the following three theories of problem causes:

- lack of a comprehensive guideline on absenteeism reduction;
- lack of compliance with the guideline on management of low-back pain by physicians;
- lack of methods to perform a strategic analysis of work and health problems in the companies.

The team found guidelines in the literature, and disseminated them among the occupational health professionals. The theories were then tested in small-scale experiments, which proved to be successful. This generated implementation of problem solutions for the entire OHS organization. Whenever problems – such as dissatisfied customers – were encountered, quality improvement teams were formed.

References

ACOEM (American College for Occupational and Environmental Medicine) (1997) *Practice Guidelines*. Beverly Farms, USA: OEM Press.

Agius, R.M. (1990) Peer review audit in occupational medicine. *J. Soc .Occup. Med.*, **40**, 87–8.

AHCPR (Agency for Health Care Policy and Research) (1995) *Using Clinical Practice Guidelines to Evaluate Quality of Care*, volume 2 *Methods*. Rockville, MD: AHCPR. Pub 95–0046.

Berwick, D.M., Godfrey, A.B. and Roessner, J. (1990) *Curing Health Care, New Strategies for Quality Improvement*. San Francisco: Jossey–Bass Inc.

Bigos, S., Bowyer, O., Braen, G. *et al.* (1994) *Acute Low Back Problems in Adults. Clinical Practice Guideline, Quick Reference Guide Number 14*. Rockville, MD: Agency for Health Care Policy and Research.

Black, N. (1996) Why we need observational studies to evaluate the effectiveness of health care. *Br. Med. J.*, **312**, 1215–18.

Bosma, Y., Verbeek, J.H.A.M. and van der Weide, W.E. (1996) Satisfactie van werknemers en bedrijfsartsen met het verzuimconsult. *Tijdschr. Bedr. Verzekerings.*, **4**, 42–8 (in Dutch).

Carey, R.G. and Lloyd, R.C. (1997) *Quality with Confidence, a Practical Guide to Quality Improvement in Healthcare*. Chicago: SPSS Inc.

Cook, T.D. and Campbell, D.T. (1979) *Quasi-Experimentation. Design and Analysis Issues for*

Field Settings. Boston, MA: Houghton Mifflin.

Daltroy, L.H., Iversen, M.D., Larson, M.G. *et al.* (1997) A controlled trial of an educational program to prevent low back injuries. *N. Engl. J. Med.*, **337**, 322–8.

Davies, H.T. and Crombie, I.K. (1995) Assessing the quality of care. *Br. Med. J.*, **311**, 766.

Donabedian, A. (1988) The quality of care. How can it be assessed? *JAMA*, **260**, 1743–48.

Draaisma, D., de Winter C.R., Dam J. *et al.* (1991). *Quality andEeffectiveness of Occupational Health Care.* The Hague: Ministry of Social Affairs and Employment (in Dutch).

Faculty of Occupational Medicine (1995) *Quality and Audit in Occupational Health.* London: Faculty of Occupational Medicine.

Grimshaw, J.M. and Russell, I.T. (1993) The effect of clinical guidelines on medical practice: a systematic review of rigorous evaluations. *Lancet*, **342**, 1317–22.

Grol, R. (1993) Development of guidelines for general practice care. *Br. J. Gen. Pract.* **43**, 146–51.

Hulshof, C.T.J., Verbeek, J.H.A.M., van Dijk, F.J.H. *et al.* (1998) How well are we doing? Evaluation research in OHS, a systematic review of empirical studies. In: *Prevention and Control of Adverse Effects of Whole-body Vibration, an Evaluation Study in Occupational Health Services* (C.T.J. Hulshof, ed.). Amsterdam: Academic thesis, University of Amsterdam, pp 73–103.

ISO (1991). *ISO 9000 International Standards for Quality Management,* 2nd edn. Geneva: ISO Central Secretariat.

de Kort, W.L.A.M., Post-Uiterweer, H.W. and van Dijk, F.J.H. (1992) Agreement on medical fitness for a job. *Scand. J. Work. Environ. Hlth*, **18**, 246–51.

Malimivaara, A., Hakkinen, U., Aro, T. *et al.* (1995) The treatment of acute low-back pain: bed rest, exercises, or ordinary activity? *N. Engl. J. Med.*, **332**, 351–5.

Meinert, C.L. (ed.) (1986) *Clinical Trials, Design, Conduct and Analysis.* New York: Oxford University Press.

Oxman, A.D. (1994) Preparing and maintaining systematic reviews. In: *Cochrane Collaboration Handbook* (A.D. Oxman, ed.). Oxford: Cochrane Collaboration.

Petitti, D.B. (1994) *Meta-analysis, Decision Analysis, and Cost-effectiveness Analysis: Methods for Quantitative Synthesis in Medicine.* New York: Oxford University Press.

Pransky, G. and Himmelstein, J. (1996) Outcomes research: implications for occupational health. *Am. J. Ind. Med.*, **29**, 573–83.

Sackett, D.L., Richardson, W.S., Rosenberg, W.M. *et al.* (1997) *Evidence-based Medicine: How to Practice and Teach EBM.* New York: Churchill Livingstone.

van der Weide, W.E., Verbeek, J.H.A.M. and van Tulder, M.W. (1997a) Vocational outcome of interventions for low-back pain. *Scand. J. Work. Environ. Hlth*, **23**, 165–178.

van der Weide, W.E., Verbeek, J.H.A.M.,van Dijk, F.J.H. *et al.* (1997b) An audit of occupational health care for employees with low-back pain. *Occup. Med.*, **47**, 294–300.

van der Weide, W.E., Verbeek, J.H.A.M., van Dijk, F.J.H. *et al.* (1998a) The development and evaluation of a quality assessment instrument for occupational physicians. *Occup. Environ. Med.*, **55**, 375–82.

van der Weide, W.E., Verbeek, J.H.A.M. and van Dijk, F.J.H. (1998b) A randomised trial of occupational rehabilitation for low-back pain. Efficacy on pain, functional disability, general health and sick leave. In: *Quality of Occupational Rehabilitation for Low-Back Pain* (W.E. van der Weide, ed.). Amsterdam: Academic Thesis, University of Amsterdam, pp. 85–99.

Wensing, M. and Grol, R. (1994) Single and combined strategies for implementing changes in primary care: a literature review. *Int. J. Quality in Health Care*, **6**, 115–32.

4

Evaluating occupational health interventions

John Øvretveit

The aim of this chapter is to help occupational health professionals better to understand an evaluation report and carry out an evaluation of their own. It presents a framework and concepts which help to analyse and design an evaluation. On the basis of these, five different evaluation designs – varying with regard to their proximity to the scientific or experimentalist ideal – are presented, in a pedagogic manner, in the form of evaluation diagrams. It is shown that a variety of designs can be used for self-review and for special research purposes in the occupational health arena. Useful evaluations do not always have to ensure control of the many variables that affect outcomes.

Nature of evaluation in an occupational health setting

Occupational health has always played an important role in protecting and promoting the health of employees and their families. But how important? And in particular, are the results worth the costs? These questions are increasingly being raised by employers and by private and social insurance services. Can particular interventions increase profitability, reduce risks, or reduce the social welfare costs of occupational diseases and accidents?

What is occupational health evaluation?

Occupational health evaluation is the attributing of value to an occupational health intervention by gathering reliable and valid information about it in a systematic way, and by making comparisons, for the purposes of making more informed decisions or understanding causal mechanisms (Øvretveit, 1998).

Financial considerations provide one reason for evaluating occupational health interventions. Two other reasons are professional and scientific. Occupational health practitioners need to review and evaluate their interventions as part of their professional work, and to develop as professionals. While this does not require specialized skills in evaluation, professional practice and development do require some knowledge of evaluation principles, and management is increasingly expecting more

sophisticated reports and assessments of occupational health programmes. Funding of occupational health services (OHS) increasingly
depends on those services providing routine evidence not only of effectiveness but also specifically of cost effectiveness.

Future programme funding increasingly depends on being able to cite
evidence of the effectiveness of a programme elsewhere and to judge the
relevance of an evaluation report to a particular organization. Willingness and ability to self-evaluate are important to the reputation of an
occupation and its position and role within an organization. Evaluation
principles and concepts improve the management of occupational health
programmes.

Evaluation studies are also required to develop the scientific disciplinary base of occupational health. We know surprisingly little about which
interventions work best in different settings, and about the factors that
account for relative success or failure. Occupational health cannot
become an evidence-based practice without a research evidence base for
practitioners to consult in deciding which intervention to make and how
to adapt it to local circumstances.

The increasing need for evaluation in and of occupational health does
not alter the fact that it is difficult to carry out even a small-scale
evaluation. Nor does it change the reality that many practitioners are not
skilled in evaluation. Many are not well-equipped to meet the demands
of evidence-based practice, or even of management, for reporting the
costs and benefits of a programme. This is not their fault – both training
and the literature on evaluation are unnecessarily complex, and rarely
use examples that are applicable to occupational health interventions
and settings. The good news is that in recent years there have been
developments in evaluation methods specifically for occupational health,
and that there is now more experience in the occupational health sector
to learn from.

The aim of this chapter is to help you to make sense of an evaluation
report and to design an evaluation study of your own. It presents designs
for simple and more complex evaluation studies that both practitioners
and researchers can use to evaluate occupational health interventions.
These designs and the basic model for drawing an evaluation will help
you quickly to read and make sense of an evaluation study. In turn, this
will help you to assess the strengths and weaknesses of an evaluation
report, and determine its implications for your practice or for occupational health policy.

Later chapters in this book refer to these designs as they are applied in
examples of evaluation research. The present chapter starts by defining
the terms we need to use to discuss evaluation, and to think about how
to evaluate a particular intervention. When starting an evaluation, what
are the first considerations? For example, 'Whom is the evaluation for?'
is one of a number of questions we need to ask at the start of any
evaluation. The chapter describes a basic model and five main types of
evaluation designs used in the occupational health arena. It describes
each design and its advantages and disadvantages. The chapter closes by
considering when and why we would use one design rather than
another.

Starting considerations

There are some basic questions to ask when reading a report of an evaluation, or when starting to design your own evaluation study. These are questions about the purpose of the evaluation. Let us take the example of an evaluation of a new general health check and screening programme for some employees. The starting questions to ask of this and of most evaluations are:

- Whom was or is the evaluation for? Who are the primary evaluation 'users'? For example, is it for the management of an organization, for an employees' union, for government policy-makers, or for other occupational health practitioners?
- Which questions does it aim to answer? For example, what are the effects of the intervention on health? Is the cost of the intervention worth the benefits?
- Which decisions and actions should be better informed as a result? What do people need to know to act differently, or to do with more confidence what they do now? For example, how do you decide whether to continue a programme, or to extend it to others?
- How do you design your own evaluation? How much time and resources are available? When are the results required? How much of your own and others' time is available? Which other resources, such as computer software or access to statistical expertise, do you need?

Other starting questions include:

- Which perspective should be taken to assess the value of the occupational health intervention? Is it just the perspective of the owners of the organization, the perspective of employees, or the perspective of the community? The more perspectives included, then the more expensive and complicated the evaluation will be.
- What are the key criteria of valuation by which the users of the evaluation will judge the value of the intervention? What is important to people? In this case, for example, how much time does the health check and screening programme take for each person. Do people do it in work-time, how much does it cost and what are its effects on health?

The language of evaluation – basic terms and concepts

The language of evaluation is essential to discussion of different designs. We have already used the most important term and concept – 'intervention'. The purpose of occupational health is to protect or improve the health of people in work settings. We aim to make a difference, i.e. to alter the course of events from what it would otherwise have been. The action involved may be a training programme, it may the enforcement of a policy or law, or it may be the provision of direct treatment (such as an influenza immunization programme). If our actions are successful, people's health will be better than it would have been if we had not. We aim to inter-vene (*inter venire*), that is, 'come between' what would otherwise have happened.

We regard the occupational health action as an intervention, even though the purpose of the evaluation is often to find out if it was in fact an intervention. Did the action actually 'inter-vene' and alter the course of events? This is especially important in an experimental design, where we consider the occupational health action as an experiment. We predict the effects of the action, and collect evidence to find out if our predictions were justified.

The main point is that we call the thing that we evaluate an 'intervention'. Later we will draw the intervention in the shape of a box, and show people being exposed to the intervention as they move through the box. A further point is that we use many different types of interventions to achieve our objectives of health protection and improvement. Occupational health physicians and nurses use treatments and diagnostic methods on an individual patient. Many interventions, however, are designed to enforce or implement policies or procedures for health (such as safety or no-smoking policies). There are also occupational health services of different kinds. They include advisory and consultation services, where the practitioner shows employers or employees how to reduce accidents or illness, or how to promote health. These are very different types of intervention.

Nevertheless, most occupational health interventions are of one of four types:

- a treatment intervention;
- a health service to a group;
- a policy or procedure;
- an indirect intervention (such as an educational programme training other people to act so as to protect or improve the health of employees).

Each of these types of intervention has a 'target', i.e. the person, population or organization which the intervention aims to affect. In sum, the key terms are (Øvretveit, 1998):

- **users** – those who make use of or act on the evaluation;
- **intervention** – an action on, or attempt to change a person, population or organization, which is the subject of an evaluation;
- **target** – the part or whole of a person, population or organization which the intervention aims to affect;
- **outcome** – the consequences of the intervention – that which 'comes out' of it;
- **target-outcome** – the change effected by the intervention on the target, i.e. the difference which the intervention makes to the target, whether intended or not;
- **'the box'** – the boundary we draw around the evaluated to define what it is we will evaluate (included in the box is a specification of the key features of the intervention);
- **dependent variable** – one of the effects we think might depend on the intervention (the outcome);

- **independent variable** – a factor that might explain the outcome, what statisticians call anything they want to assess for its possible effect on the outcome (e.g. being a member of an experimental group);
- **control group** – a group of people who do not get the intervention;
- **retrospective evaluation** – looking into the past for evidence about the intervention (by contrast with 'concurrent', meaning at the same time);
- **prospective evaluation** – designing an evaluation and then collecting data while the intervention is happening, and usually also before and after the intervention;
- **criteria** – the comparisons against which we judge the evaluated (effectiveness is often one such criterion);
- **operationalize** – converting something general (e.g. a criterion) into something specific, usually into something that we can measure;
- **outcome measure** – a measure of an important predicted effect of the intervention on the target person or population (e.g. a measure of amount of sleep, or of how long awake).

Drawing an evaluation design – the basic model

One of the quickest ways to make sense of an evaluation, or to design one, is to draw a diagram of it. The diagram shows the intervention – such as a health-screening programme – inside 'the box', and people being exposed to the intervention as 'passing through' the box. Usually we examine the effect the intervention has – the difference it makes – and concentrate on the predicted or intended difference. In our example, the people receiving the health screening should be different in that they will know more about their health. The organization should be different in now having more knowledge of the health of its employees, as well as now having fewer resources – the screening programme having consumed resources that could have been used for other purposes. In experimental evaluations, we predict the difference and then measure to discover if the prediction was fulfilled.

Figure 4.1 shows the intervention to be evaluated inside a 'box'. This 'box' represents the occupational health treatment, service, policy or organizational change to be evaluated. The 'box boundary' defines what

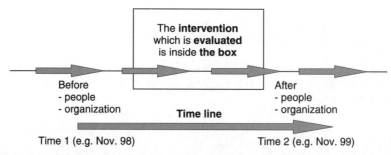

Figure 4.1 *The basic drawing of an evaluation design: if you cannot draw it, then it is not clear or understood*

is and is not evaluated. Accordingly, if we were evaluating a no-smoking policy at work we would write 'no-smoking policy' in the box. We would consider other things happening during the same period, such as a redundancy programme, as changes that are not to be evaluated and as being outside the box. Such other changes might affect the measures we use of peoples' health when we look at people before and after. Later we will consider how we can take account of other factors that might confuse our evaluation of the intervention (termed 'confounders').

In what follows, this basic diagram is used to show five different types of evaluation designs commonly used to evaluate occupational health interventions. When looking through these, consider which is the best design for evaluating an employee health screening programme. Remember that there is no single best design, only one that is feasible given the resources available, and most suited to the purposes of the evaluation. This is the one that best answers users' questions and helps them make more informed decisions.

Type 1 design – descriptive

The purpose of the evaluation design depicted in Figure 4.2 is to produce a description of the intervention being evaluated, and also a description of 'important' features of the 'environment' surrounding the intervention, so as to enable users to make a more informed judgement of the value of the intervention. The design does not measure outcomes. Typical questions answered by this design are 'What is it?' and 'What happens?'

Sometimes, a descriptive evaluation is needed by managers who are remote from what is happening and who ask for an evaluation. After discussion, it becomes apparent that they do not have the time or money for an outcome evaluation and actually only want a description of 'what is really happening' by an independent observer. Another reason for

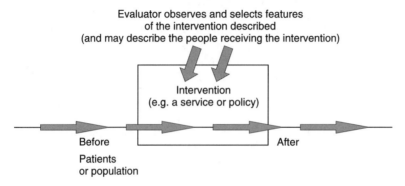

Figure 4.2 *Design type 1 – descriptive*

performing a descriptive evaluation of an existing programme or policy is to give a precise description that allows other people to set up a similar programme or to carry out a similar policy. Also, it may be premature to try to judge the value of something if there is not an agreed and explicit description of it, which is the case with some occupational health interventions.

In the example of a health-screening programme, the evaluation would simply describe the programme and what was done. Note that the evaluator does not just observe and describe, but is influenced by concepts and theories to decide what to describe and how to conceptualize the intervention. The description would probably note features of the organization which helped and hindered setting up and running the programme (i.e. the intervention context) and any changes that were introduced to the programme over time. A descriptive design might also be appropriate to describe a change to how an organization works that is thought to have had an impact on employees' health, but where there is some uncertainty as to exactly what was changed. In this case, the change is regarded as an intervention, and the descriptive design is used just to get a good description of what the change was.

If the description uses explicit standards and criteria to decide what to describe or to compare the programme against, then it is a Type 2 audit design. If the description involves a before–after comparison, then it is a Type 3 outcome evaluation (see below).

The main strength of the Type 1 design is that it does not need many resources to carry out. It can be done in collaboration with service providers and people receiving a treatment, and can clarify objectives and highlight problems. Its weaknesses are that it can be ignored as unscientific, biased or trivial, and does not give data on effects. The usefulness of such evaluations depends on the skill, knowledge and credibility of the evaluator, and the theoretical perspective which he or she uses to select and conceptualize what to describe. For example, a descriptive evaluation by a health economist would be different to one by an anthropologist or psychologist.

Some might say that we cannot really call a simple Type 1 design an evaluation. But sometimes when people want something evaluated they are often unsure exactly what it is they want to evaluate, what the aims of the evaluation are, or what questions they want answered (i.e. what is in 'the box'). Evaluators can be only too ready to propose a sophisticated and expensive design when more consideration of the user's concerns and questions would show that all that is needed is an independent description, which then helps to judge value.

Descriptive evaluations can be used to describe a new or unfamiliar occupational health programme or policy, but are more often employed to describe a service or policy that is unclear or in the early stages of evolution. Descriptive evaluations may or may not describe the costs of an intervention. They can be 'retrospective' – done after a change or a policy is carried out (e.g. many 'summative' evaluations), or 'concurrent' – done while a policy is being implemented (e.g. many 'developmental' or 'formative' evaluations).

Type 2 design – audit

The design in Figure 4.3 is used for inspection, compliance monitoring, managerial monitoring of policy implementation, simple economic audits, developmental self- or peer review exercises, and some types of quality assurance and clinical audit. The question it is designed to answer is 'Did the intervention follow procedures or achieve the objectives set for it?' The purpose of the design is to judge the value of what people are doing by comparing what they do with what they are supposed to do.

This design is like a Type 1 evaluation, but describes the occupational health intervention or policy in comparison with intended objectives, procedures, standards or norms (which are usually specified in writing). The audit may be carried out by external evaluators or by the organization itself using established standards. One weakness of the design is that it depends on having a clearly specified set of standards, procedures or objectives (e.g. a clear law or statement of policy), or on creating such a set as part of the evaluation. The design does not help to judge the value of the intervention, but just whether people 'follow orders'. Note that there is an implicit assumption that if people follow procedures then they are doing something of value, but it may be that the intervention is ineffective or inappropriate. The strengths of the design are that few resources are needed, it can be done quickly, it is good for self-evaluation, it is usually of some use, it can promote understanding of why a policy or intervention fails or succeeds, and it can sometimes give generalizable knowledge.

Audit designs assume that if service providers follow the relevant standards, then a beneficial outcome will follow. But this may not have been proven before. The evaluation design does not permit discovery of effects or possible causes, but it can be used to audit outcome or performance, e.g. show how well an employer complies with employee rights or safety standards. Checking whether practitioners are following treatment guidelines is one type of audit evaluation. However, the term 'clinical audit' also refers to clinicians first deciding which guidelines

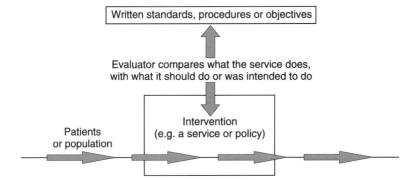

Figure 4.3 *Design type 2 – audit*

and criteria to use. Where decisions are based on evidence of effectiveness, then an audit has greater value. Other types of audit evaluations are of services, e.g. a quality assurance audit of OHS using a set of quality standards, or a policy audit to check whether people are complying with a policy. Audits may be retrospective or concurrent, and may or may not consider costs.

Some would not consider auditing to be a type of evaluation because the design does not aim to evaluate the effectiveness of an intervention. Rather, it evaluates whether people carry out procedures, achieve objectives, or meet standards. 'Monitoring' is certainly a better term to describe many of the activities encompassed by this design, but here we are taking a broad view of evaluation and auditing deserves to be included as one of its forms. One particular reason for so doing is that information about whether people or services meet specifications or objectives is an increasingly important way of judging the value of what they are doing (specifications and objectives are based on evidence about what is effective). Generally, the value of an audit depends on the validity of its guidelines, standards, procedures or objectives, and whether these have been derived from evaluations carried out using other designs.

Type 3 design – before and after

The type of design shown in Figure 4.4 is used for discovering limited or broad changes in people undergoing an occupational health treatment, or which result from a new policy or change in working arrangements. It is usually employed within an experimentalist perspective where the intervention is viewed as an experiment and the evaluator predicts the effects of the intervention on certain targets. The purpose of the design is to help to judge the value of an intervention by comparing the state of people (or organizations) 'before' with their state 'after' the intervention (outcome measurement). The questions this design aims to answer are 'What are the effects of the intervention?' or 'What difference does the intervention make to the target?'

The before–after comparison may be of two single-measured states (e.g. blood pressures or stress levels), or of a number of features of the target (e.g. a set of employee perceptions, physical measures, providers'

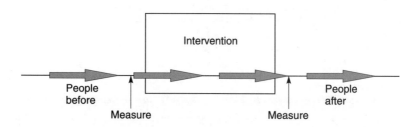

Figure 4.4 *Design type 3 – before and after*

assessments of 'patient progress', employee income losses etc.). The before–after comparisons are based on theories and predictions about the possible effects of the intervention. The main weakness of the design is that it cannot give conclusive objective evidence of effects. This is because if a before–after difference is found, it may have been caused by things other than the intervention (many possible 'confounding variables' are not controlled for). Further, the subjects selected may have shown these effects over time in any case. Its strengths are that evaluations can be small-scale and relatively quick. The design can be arranged to use few resources if the evaluator selects a small number of subjects, constructs one or a few simple 'before' and 'after' measures, and makes the measurement soon after the intervention.

By contrast with Types 1 and 2, many would regard the Type 3 design as the first recognizable evaluation design. This is because it looks at an outcome, or rather the difference that an intervention might make to a target. However, those who take this view might also be dissatisfied with how the design tries to discover the effect of the intervention. How does it prove that the difference is due to the intervention and not to something else? Would there have been a difference even without the intervention?

The diagram in Figure 4.4 can be misleading for some types of evaluation where the treatment or intervention does not stop. The drawing shows that people 'pass through' an intervention and are then no longer exposed to it. Sometimes, people continue to be treated or to receive the service. Examples include medication for hypertension, interventions for chronic disorders, and home care services. For these people, the diagram shows that a measure is taken before they start and then at periods after first receiving the treatment.

Type 4 design – comparative

One of the questions addressed by the design in Figure 4.5 is 'What are the effects of the intervention compared with a similar intervention or with the status quo elsewhere?' The design might be used for economic and quasi-experimental evaluation of two different employment policies, or for an evaluation of different types of OHS. Further, it could be used to evaluate a training programme compared with a written-information intervention, or to compare two or more different treatments.

The design is like a Type 3 outcome evaluation, but compares the outcomes of two groups undergoing different interventions. Variations include a retrospective design (e.g. some comparative evaluations of different policies or work conditions) and comparison of end-states only (rather than a comparison of before–after change).

The weaknesses of the design are that it is expensive, and that it is difficult to prove that effects are due to interventions alone rather than other factors. The main strength is that, with careful design, such evaluations can suggest which of two interventions is more effective or cost-effective. The design is suitable where it is unethical or impractical to treat or intervene in only one group.

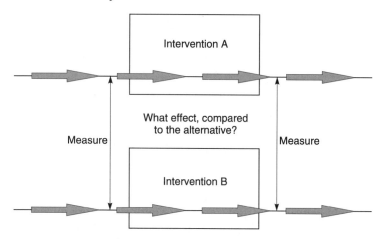

Figure 4.5 *Design type 4 – comparative*

Unlike Type 3 designs, this design compares two interventions, but it does make use of a Type 3 before–after outcome comparison. It is a common design for evaluations of treatments or services, e.g. where a new treatment or service is started on one site, which people want to compare with a traditional treatment or service on another site. Possible concrete examples are a comparison of the health states of patients before and after a new rehabilitation technique, and comparing a service for stroke patients with conventional rehabilitation. Evaluations of this kind are often carried out according to experimental principles ('controlled trials'). They have hypotheses to test and different methods for controlling for influences other than the interventions, such as patient characteristics (e.g. age, sex, severity of illness, duration of previous illness etc.). A common control technique is to 'match' the characteristics of the people experiencing each intervention. The aim of matching is to try to exclude influences that might affect the outcome other than the intervention, but matching is less good for this purpose than random allocation (see the Type 5 design below).

The Type 4 design, like the Type 3 design, can be used when conditions allow a 'natural experiment'. One example is the performing of a retrospective evaluation where there are records or measures already available. Within the experimental perspective, however, prospective designs are preferred because this allows the evaluator to arrange beforehand for better experimental controls and more rigorous hypothesis testing.

Comparative-outcome evaluations of this type can give some objective evidence of the effect of the intervention compared with another one, but they take longer and use more resources than Type 3 designs. The cost and resource time required increase with more subjects (which calls for more time and care in matching subjects), with more complex measures (e.g. quality-of-life measures), with more than one 'after' measure, and with longer intervening periods between intervention and measurement.

The essential difference between the Type 4 and the Type 3 designs is that the former compares two interventions, and the difference to Type 5 is that people are not randomly allocated. Further, in Type 4, one of the interventions is not a placebo; accordingly, controls are fewer than in the case of the Type 5, full experimental design.

Type 5 design – randomized control

This is the 'classic' evaluation design (Figure 4.6), which many think of as the 'proper' evaluation of a treatment or a service. Its idea is to create two groups that are exactly the same in all respects apart from the fact that one group received the intervention. The design can rule out many alternative explanations for a change that is detected in the targets, and can give evidence of causal mechanisms. Its purpose is to compare the effects of an intervention on one group compared with that on another group which does not get the intervention, but who are in all other possible respects similar. The design addresses the question of the effects of an intervention on an experimental compared with a control group. It is used to gain 'conclusive' evidence of the effect of a treatment or service on one or a few measures of the health state of a group of patients.

The design is like the Type 4 design, but the people selected for the intervention are randomly assigned to a control (placebo) and an intervention group. This design is capable of reducing the number of possible explanations for any differences between outcomes for the two groups being due to things other than the intervention (the 'randomized controlled trial'). The control group do not simply 'get nothing', but receive an intervention called a 'placebo'. Some estimates suggest that 30–40% of patients will show an improvement without intervention. In the occupational health arena, however, it may be quite difficult to arrange a placebo, and this can reduce the validity of the design.

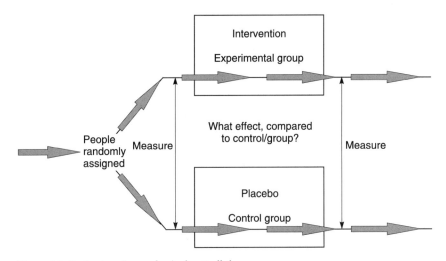

Figure 4.6 *Design type 5 – randomized controlled*

The weaknesses of the design are that it is expensive, takes time and needs evaluators with experience, skill and statistical expertise to produce credible results. Often, evaluations of this design do not take account of patients' subjective experiences, and the group average may mask extreme effects on some individuals. The design has been criticized as not allowing generalization of findings to normal settings because it uses careful selection of subjects (to maximize controls) that are not typical. The design maximizes 'internal' validity at the expense of 'external' validity. Nine other criticisms are listed by Øvretveit (1998). Strengths are that the design gives more reliable and valid information about the effect of an intervention than Type 3 simple outcome evaluation, and Type 4 non-random, non-placebo comparison. Results of a well-conducted evaluation of this design usually have high credibility among clinicians.

The design can be retrospective, but – when looking back over time – it is usually difficult to get a good control group or to check whether the intervention was stable. Type 5 designs are usually prospective. They are called 'experimental' because the evaluator intervenes to create a change, and then studies it using principles and controls similar to those employed by a natural scientist in a laboratory.

The full design is not suitable for evaluating many occupational health interventions because of difficulties in controlling for extraneous variables, and even in controlling the intervention itself. Whether it should be regarded as the ideal design from which the occupational health evaluator reluctantly diverges is another matter. But, for some interventions – such as many concerned with diagnosis or treatment – there is no doubt that it can be the best for answering certain questions, always provided that resources and time are available.

Concluding remarks

To understand an evaluation report, and to decide upon a design, it helps to draw a diagram with:

- a 'box' around what was evaluated (the intervention);
- any 'before' and 'after' measures, and when they were taken;
- the timescale, and the number of people involved.

When reading an evaluation report, or when planning your own evaluation, the first thing to do is to define what was or is to be evaluated – 'What is the intervention?', 'What is to be put "in the box"?'. If you are not exactly sure what was evaluated in a study, then you cannot understand the study. This may be because the evaluated was badly described, or because it was a poor study that did not define the intervention evaluated. In planning an evaluation of your own, you will need to specify clearly the 'thing' – the policy/process – that you are to evaluate before you start. The diagram forces you to think about what is 'in the box' and what is not.

The five diagrams of evaluation designs are useful for people new to evaluation to see some of the different types that are possible. It is helpful when reading an evaluation report to try to draw it in this way – to draw the 'box' and the type of design to show the essential features. Most evaluations use one of five types of designs:

- **descriptive** – a description of features of the intervention or implementation process;
- **audit** – a comparison of what is done in relation to specified standards or objectives;
- **outcome** – the 'before' state of the target of an intervention compared with its 'after' state;
- **comparative** – a comparison of the 'before' and 'after' states of people receiving two or more different interventions;
- **randomized-control** – a comparison of a defined 'before' and 'after' state between people randomly allocated to an intervention and a placebo group.

Different designs answer different questions, and some designs are more expensive and take longer than others. Whether the extra time and cost is worth it depends on the particular questions addressed and for whom the evaluation is being performed. An evaluation does not need to be an experimental randomized-control trial or have a comparative design for it to be useful. Much depends on whom the evaluation is for, their questions and their valuation criteria. A randomized control trial may be too expensive, take too long for some users, and may not be practical or even ethical.

Evaluations are designed to help people make better informed decisions than they would otherwise do. However, for inexpert users who cannot assess study limitations, a poorly designed and conducted evaluation is worse than none at all. It may be misleading rather than informative.

There is considerable debate about whether the experimentalist approach to evaluation is the best or even only approach. In the occupational health arena, we need to adopt different approaches for different interventions. Action evaluation and qualitative data-gathering will be necessary for some. Occupation health can learn much from recent work in the health-promotion field about methods for evaluation other than the traditional experimentalist (Macdonald *et al.*, 1996). However, the experimentalist approach does emphasize ideas fundamental to many types of evaluation – an operational measure of outcome, a hypothesis about what produces the outcome, being open-minded about anything that might affect the outcome, and the idea of control (of the intervention, and of things other than the intervention that might vary).

Details of design and data gathering depend on:

- the subject of the evaluation – whether the intervention is a treatment, a service, a policy or organizational intervention;
- the target of the intervention – a person, a population of employees, or employees and their families;
- the purpose of the intervention and questions to be answered – to decide whether it works, how and why it works, whether it is worth the money, how to make it better, how well it performs;

- the users of the evaluation – managers, clinicians, patients, policy-makers, the public as payer, other scientists/researchers;
- the evaluation perspective – experimental, economic, developmental, or managerial;
- the methods for gathering and analysing data within the broad categories of quantitative or qualitative methods.

Considerations in designing an evaluation include:

- which user perspective(s) to take;
- which decisions and actions could be informed by the evaluation (What do people need to know to act differently, or to do with more confidence what they do now?);
- users' criteria of valuation;
- criteria of comparison to be used in the evaluation;
- the questions the evaluation aims to answer.

References

Øvretveit, J. (1998) *Evaluating Health Interventions*. Milton Keynes: Open University Press.

Macdonald, G., Veen, C. and Tones, K. (1996) Evidence for success in health promotion: suggestions for improvement. *Hlth Educ. Res.*, **11**(3), 367-76.

5

Quantitative methods in medical audit for OHS evaluation

Raymond Agius, Robert Lee, Gillian Fletcher and Joanna Uttley

This chapter considers the variety of purposes of the medical audit, and in particular the quantitative methods that may be appropriate for assuring quality through the auditing of occupational health services (OHS). The procedure is illustrated with real examples based on research, and on internal or external peer reviews, thereby indicating some ways forward and possible solutions. A contrast is made between quantitative research and audit, and the need for evidence-based approaches is highlighted.

Quantitative methods for evaluation and quality assurance may serve a number of purposes:

- to determine, as part of a formative assessment, the effectiveness and efficiency of an OHS organization as a whole;
- to determine the need for change, e.g. in policy and in other planning, and to evaluate any changes implemented;
- to evaluate the contribution of health care professionals, and hence to help identify and plan education, training or other interventions;
- to determine compliance with a standard, or with a service level agreement in terms of the structure of services, the quality of their processes and/or the effectiveness of their outcome;
- in so doing, to aid communication and find gaps in the evidence base for current practice, thus setting the agenda for further research, evaluation and hence wider improvements in quality.

Terminology and taxonomy

Some terms used in this chapter are defined below, since they might have different meanings elsewhere in this book.

To **evaluate** is defined by the *Concise Oxford Dictionary* as 'to ascertain the amount of', 'to find numerical expression for', 'to appraise, assess'. In the context of this work, evaluation may be interpreted as a quantitative assessment comparing the contribution of a service or activity or intervention with the situation existing before or elsewhere. In other words, in evaluation a quantitative comparison is made with a prior situation or an external control, whereas in the context of audit, a comparison is usually made specifically with a criterion-based standard.

In occupational health, as in other branches of health care, audit can be classified into Donabedian's three categories of structure, process and outcome.

The terms **clinical audit** and **medical audit** are used to describe the systematic criterion-based review of the work of health professionals. Different countries or languages may vary in their understanding of what these terms encompass. However, as far as possible, audit should be inclusive of all professional groups within OHS, and other staff in the workplace should be included in its non-confidential aspects.

The origin of the word audit lies in the Latin *audire*, 'to listen'. Accordingly, the activity has to be based on a process of consultation – in this context where managers, employees, occupational physicians, other health professionals and auditors (external or internal) are partners. Audit can be conducted internally for the purposes of improving quality of care and to assist in education, or it may be conducted by outsiders as part of a quality certification process, or to ensure compliance with a pre-determined level of service.

Assessing needs

In order to achieve an efficient and effective occupational health service, quantitative evaluation and audit must themselves be effective and efficient. Using qualitative methods, it is essential to identify important or problematic areas and to establish priorities among them. Some important principles need to be borne in mind to ensure the relevance and validity of plans for any quantitative assessment, such as audit. These are shown in Box 5.1.

Box 5.1 Important principles in planning quantitative evaluation and audit

- Audit the validity of policies on epidemiological grounds rather than whether the policies simply exist or not.
- Audit critical stages in the activity, e.g. assessing control measures and identification of all employees at significant risk, before auditing less critical aspects such as the exact times when workers are assessed.
- Focus on the more crucial aspects of the process, e.g. the sensitivity, specificity, reliability of questions in the clinical assessment, before less crucial tools but which may be easier to audit (e.g. the accuracy of lung function equipment).
- Audit the quality of occupational health responses (in terms of predictive value or eventual prognostic validity) and not merely the frequency of their activity or the punctuality of the response to management referrals.

Needs assessments for OHS can form the basis of service level agreements for occupational health which consistently cover all workers wherever they may be located. These agreements in turn can incorporate criteria of quality and service that are amenable to audit. Throughout, the aim is to provide the same high standard of care and high-quality advice to management and employees, and thus promote a high standard of health and safety at work (see Box 5.2).

Box 5.2 Needs assessment for OHS delivery, followed by quantitative audit programme

An organization within the health care industry reviewed the provision of its OHS. A representative sample of all employees in terms of age, sex, seniority, managerial responsibility and trade union involvement were interviewed in a semi-structured manner. Additional information was gathered from managers and through site visits by OH specialists. Major risks identified included the risk of transmission of viruses to employees, the risks of sensitization, and the necessity of compliance with legal requirements.

The information gathered from these sources led to the establishment of a range of new policies, covering the full spectrum of OH activities, e.g. pre-employment health assessment, health surveillance for sensitizers, sickness absence etc. These policies were used as the basis of service level agreements set up between management and local OH providers. Finally, the audit plan was agreed:

- **Structure:** The audit of structure compared the facilities, training, sources of information, confidential storage of health records etc. of the OH providers against the agreed standard, but was not a substantial feature of the audit.
- **Process:** Critical processes such as health surveillance were audited to ensure that they were performing sensitively and specifically in identifying work-related ill-health. A sample of the OH response in terms of the appropriateness of the reply to questions posed by management in sickness absence referrals was audited (Agius et al., 1995). A sample of records of self-referrals of employees was audited confidentially by other OH staff using agreed criteria.
- **Outcome:** Some topics were subject to an audit of outcome, e.g. by determining specific antibody levels following vaccination of employees at risk of hepatitis B.

In conclusion, some shortcomings were found when compared to the pre-agreed standard. For example discrepancies in the outcome of the vaccination programme, in health surveillance and pre-employment assessment process, and in management of self-referrals were identified. In consultation with the OH providers, steps were taken to bring about improvement, and the terms for subsequent audits were then agreed.

Quality in audit

To establish priority areas for audit, the initial focus should be on areas of high cost in terms of health, employment, or service delivery. It is only possible to identify the specific processes, outcomes or tools for audit after these priority areas have been defined. Accordingly, it may be more important to invest in targeted, valid health surveillance for those at greatest risk rather than in unnecessarily detailed pre-employment assessment for all staff. For example, auditing structure, process and outcome in relation to respiratory symptoms in the workforce might be highly relevant and critical to an electronics plant engaged in soldering using colophony, but is probably irrelevant to a bank.

There may be a tendency to audit or evaluate the activities that consume most resources (Agius et al., 1993). If these activities are validated by a needs assessment, then such an approach may help in improving both effectiveness and efficiency. However, it is very important to resist the temptation to audit what can be easily audited instead of what needs to be audited.

A procedure in which there are wide variations in observed practice is much more likely to benefit from audit against an agreed standard. If no such standard exists, then it is important to make quantitative measurements to evaluate planned interventions to promote or protect health.

External demands and expectations

Since international quality standards of the ISO-9000 type are gaining in popularity and application in industry, it is not surprising that purchasers and providers of OHS may seek their extrapolation to this sector (MacDonald et al., 1995). However, the extension of such quality-management systems to occupational health practice requires careful consideration. Again the focus should be on aspects that are crucial to occupational health care, not merely on those that can be easily measured and audited. For example, investigating the strategy for workplace air monitoring, the sensitivity and specificity of respiratory questionnaires, and the identification of at-risk workers are all vital components of health surveillance for asthmagens. Confirming the calibration of spirometers is not enough. Accordingly, certified quality management systems that do not address the scientific, epidemiological and clinical validity of OHS practice may be of limited value.

Issues of quality in occupational health must be addressed throughout the entire working organization, not merely within its OHS unit. The quality of information input to OHS might be so poor that output in terms of advice and recommendations is bound to be limited. In this context, it is as important to audit the quality of the information received as it is to audit the process by which the information is handled.

The organization's response to OHS is crucial. Thus, an audit of the management of sickness-absence referrals by an OHS unit will have limited value if it does not also address the extent to which the organization as a whole recognizes, accepts and implements appropriate referrals (Agius et al., 1995). The employing organization then needs to implement advice to prevent ill-health and to rehabilitate.

Different, and changing, models of OHS delivery also raise important issues. Free-standing OHS selling their services on a contractual basis may adopt quality-assurance (QA) approaches analogous to those of any commercial free-market undertaking (e.g. the ISO-9000 series). However, it is important that their audit should apply essential and specific clinical and epidemiological criteria to ensure the best health outcome for the specific workforce as a whole as well as for individuals within it.

Some other important reservations need to be stated. For example, if, in the course of an initial assessment, manifestly inadequate staff competencies are identified, it may be more practical to arrange further training and recruitment than to start a time-consuming and costly exercise to quantify the consequences of poor competencies. For example, a controlled trial of internal peer review audit extending over 2 years showed a significant but limited improvement in the process of medical consultations (Agius *et al.*, 1994). The difference attributable to audit was small compared with the magnitude of differences in practice attributable to the prior training of physicians. This suggests that while audit can be a useful tool to alter and improve practice, it is perhaps a poor substitute for adequate professional training.

Determining methodology

Quantitative methods are generally indispensable for the purposes of auditing an OHS organization or evaluating an occupational health intervention. However, they are often not adequate in themselves, and qualitative methods find important application in a number of areas (e.g. determining customer satisfaction). The purposes and hence the methods of evaluation vary according to the perspective of the observer (Husman, 1993).

Audit of structure, e.g. of premises, is relatively cheap and easy but might have no bearing whatever on the effectiveness and efficiency of OHS.

Audit of process can be very valuable if it addresses important determinants of outcome, and has many advantages (Crombie and Davies, 1998). It can be cheaper, more sensitive and permit quicker remedial actions than audit of outcome. In occupational health practice too, the ultimate goal may need to be evaluated through various intermediary steps or 'outputs' – for example, the advice given by OHS to managers (Agius *et al.*, 1995; van der Weide *et al.*, 1998).

Audit of outcome intuitively appears more valuable than audit of process but it may entail high expense and require a longer time scale, especially if a demonstrable reduction in health risk is taken as an outcome standard.

Ill-health outcome in a workplace is not synonymous with the quality of output of the service delivered, since the occupational health and safety 'outcome' for workers is not independently determined by the quality of the OHS. The attitude and commitment of managers, as well as the level of communication between workforce and employers, is often the limiting factor. Methods are being developed to implement a wide range of audits in OHS (MacDonald *et al.*, 1995), but – whatever the approach – it should take certain specific steps (see Box 5.3 below).

Quantitative methods are still imperfect, and their application should help in determining gaps in the evidence base for current practice and shortcomings in methodology. Hence, they may assist in setting the agenda for further research.

Box 5.3 Implementing quantitative evaluation and audit

- Review the evidence base for the relevant area(s).
- Debate and agree practice guidelines for the above.
- Educate practitioners in the implementation of the practice guidelines.
- Develop audit criteria based on the practice guidelines.
- Audit a representative sample of practice against the audit criteria.
- Implement change, and close the loop.

Setting criteria and standards

The audit 'cycle' involves comparing observed practice with a set standard, followed by appropriate improvement. However, there may be no 'gold standard' and an initial 'audit' might consist simply of observing practice, measuring the variation in practice, and thence debating and researching an appropriate standard (Agius *et al.*, 1993).

A standard should ideally be set on the basis of good original research or a review of research conducted by others – as in Cochrane collaborations. Setting a standard based on current practice may be flawed if it merely reflects a majority or dominant view, or just tradition. Inadequate evidence-based standards of practice in occupational health constitute a fundamental weakness. In many contexts, it has been shown that there is a wide diversity of practice between different OHS organizations, and also between different categories of occupational health practitioners ostensibly working to achieve the same end (Whitaker and Aw, 1995).

In setting standards by which to audit, it is important – as far as feasible – to set explicit criteria with detailed definitions rather than loose guidelines (van der Weide *et al.*, 1998). They should be such that the audit can be reliably carried out by persons, following training, other than those who agreed on the standards. This does not mean that the standards will be immutable – but reasons for departing from them must be noted and form the basis for further debate and revision. Local adaptations of standards, if properly evaluated, may later find a wider application.

Research has addressed only a fraction of OHS practice. A fundamental difficulty lies in setting criteria and standards for the application of quantitative methods (Agius *et al.*, 1993; van der Weide *et al.*, 1997, 1998) to the audit and evaluation of changes in services delivered. For most occupational health practitioners therefore, the most pressing demand is to adopt a practical approach to the setting of criteria and standards. The steps for this are summarized in Box 5.4.

Box 5.4 Essential steps in improving quality of OH practice

- Determine research needs – by systematically debating and reviewing existing practice, especially if high cost implications in terms of health, employment, or service delivery.
- Commission and conduct the necessary research and/or
- Commission and conduct systematic reviews of the Cochrane type.
- Train and educate on the basis of the systematic reviews.
- Audit a sample of OH practice against the reviewed standard.
- Implement change and close the loop.

An example of setting standards and audit criteria illustrated by the problem of respiratory sensitization is shown in Box 5.5. The table includes only a small part of the stages in the management of respiratory sensitization, and a more detailed account can be found elsewhere (Agius, 1995).

Box 5.5 From research evidence to audit criteria – an example

Scientific evidence	Practice guidelines	Audit criteria indicating non-compliance
Atopy *per se* has poor predictive value in relation to pre-employment assessment.	Applicants exposed to respiratory sensitizers should not be excluded on the basis of atopy alone.	Policy or practice of excluding employee(s) on the basis of atopy alone.
Questionnaires including (specified) questions on respiratory symptoms and applied at a defined frequency are a sensitive way of identifying occupational asthma.	Specification of questions to be included in questionnaire. Frequency and mode of administration of questionnaire.	Policy or practice not using a valid questionnaire (in terms of sensitivity etc.).
Specificity can then be achieved through other (defined) ways, e.g. lung function tests before and after exposure.	Protocol for further investigation using spirometry, workplace assessment etc.	Positive responses not followed up using appropriate specific investigations.

Comparing observations with standards

Whether the audit addresses process or outcome, it should be comprehensive and ensure that all clinical encounters or outcome parameters, occupational-hygiene reports, and so on are available. All this constitutes the sampling frame. A sample of these data should be selected at random, though a larger sample may be appropriate for higher risk/cost situations. All aspects of the audit topic should be available for comparison with the set standard.

Audit has investigated variation in process and output in relation to resource-intensive practices within large organizations. In the health service, an audit of pre-employment assessment revealed wide variations in process (Whitaker *et al.*, 1995). This provided evidence to question the policy of and the evidence for pre-employment screening, with the goal of improving its effectiveness and efficiency. Even when good scientific evidence of the value of certain procedures is available, they may be ignored in practice. Guidance on suitable topics for audit and some detailed accounts of audits – of, for example, sickness absence and back pain – are available in published materials (Seaton *et al.*, 1994; Agius *et al.*, 1995; van der Weide *et al.*, 1997, 1998).

Conventional epidemiological methods can be used to conduct pre- and post-intervention evaluations, e.g. by measuring prevalence of symptoms of musculoskeletal pain before and after ergonomic interventions (Westerholm, 1995). Qualitative and quantitative methods can address

---

Box 5.6 Audit of back pain assessments (n = 35)

	Satisfactorily recorded items	Percentage satisfactory out of relevant denominator (not always 35)
History		
Timing of onset	34	97
Symptomatic description	29	83
Pain aggravation/tolerance	26	74
Past history	29	83
Examination		
Pain distribution	23	66
Local back signs	20	57
Straight leg raising	21	62
Diagnosis/conclusions		
Anatomic/pathologic/ aetiologic	18	53
Objective impairment	15	44
Advice/action		
Work fitness	34	97
Rehabilitation	11	31

This audit showed that while the clinical history taking was generally satisfactory in these consultations, physical examination, a diagnostic conclusion and an explicit statement of physical impairment was less frequent. Conclusions on fitness for work were almost universal but rehabilitation could have been more thoroughly pursued. These data can suggest the need for improved policies, training and practice in rehabilitation in the workplace.

occupational health interactions between managers/employers and employees, such as with regard to the quality of management referrals (Agius *et al.*, 1995) or of communication between relevant parties. This should lead to joint initiatives to audit the response to occupational health advice, e.g. on prevention of ill-health and rehabilitation.

Within OHS units themselves, the need for a range of disciplinary skills needs consideration, since most issues demand a team approach. An internal audit group is possible, and may be formed among occupational health professionals from different disciplines or levels of expertise (especially for educational purposes) by members taking turns in the role of auditors.

Clinical assessment of specific problems is an important part of occupational health practice, e.g. in relation to common problems such as back pain and other musculoskeletal disorders. Comparison of observed practice with standards has been undertaken by van der Weide and colleagues (1997), and guidelines for this purpose have been previously published (Seaton *et al.*, 1994). For example, a random selection of OHS records of consultations in relation to back pain was audited by external peer review. A summary of the results and an interpretation of the exercise is presented in Box 5.6.

Box 5.7 Audit of respiratory assessments ($n = 20$)

	Satisfactorily recorded items	Percentage satisfactory out of relevant denominator (not always 20)
History		
Timing of onset	16	80
Drug treatment	14	73
Smoking	10	50
Exposures	16	84
Examination		
Clinical examination	15	75
Lung function test	8	53
Diagnosis/conclusions		
Nature of condition	17	85
Causative factors	12	67
Functional impairment	9	56
Advice/action		
Work fitness	14	78
Reduction of exposure	4	50

This audit suggested that there were generally good records in relation to the timing of onset and the description of the symptoms, but smoking habits were not consistently noted. Moreover objective records of lung function testing and specific advice on reduction of exposure might need to be pursued more often.

Work-related respiratory ill-health is another common issue for which evidence-based criteria may be developed (see Box 5.5 above). A practical application of auditing OHS consultations relating to respiratory ill-health, conducted by external peer review is illustrated in Box 5.7.

Where work-related skin disease is a significant problem, simple questionnaires validated by inspection may be used to determine prevalence before and after implementing specific preventive measures. In the workplace described in Box 5.2 above, such an exercise was conducted following an outbreak of probable work-related dermatitis. Audit of the individual management of problems such as this is exemplified in Box 5.8.

Box 5.8 Audit of skin assessments (n = 18)

	Satisfactorily recorded items	Percentage satisfactory out of relevant denominator (not always 18)
History		
Timing of onset	12	67
Symptomatic description	14	78
Drug treatment	11	69
Exposures	13	22
Examination		
Distribution of lesions	15	88
Description of lesions	14	78
Diagnosis/conclusions		
Nature of condition	13	72
Possible causative agent(s)	10	59
Advice/action		
Work fitness	15	83
Reduction of exposure	14	78

This audit suggested generally satisfactory case assessment and management, but the relatively low proportion of definitive causal diagnoses prompts a debate as to the need for more specialist investigation, and perhaps patch testing.

In many situations, evaluation will be very important because of the frequency of a problem, and its perceived significance. Yet, in the case of mental health conditions, much ill-health is hidden. In many instances, it manifests itself in confidential self-referral, which may be handled by a wide range of occupational health practitioners and methods.

Various approaches to auditing the self-referred component of OHS work may be adopted, although probably no one method alone is ideal. A systematic peer reviewed audit of OHS practice can provide the basis for debate, further education, and perhaps policy changes – though not necessarily a prescriptive solution (as illustrated in Box 5.9 below).

Moreover, a summary of audit findings without identifying individuals can demonstrate to managers or user groups that self-referred problems are being addressed satisfactorily by OHS, as judged by professional peer review, but that some issues may need to be tackled at an organizational level.

Box 5.9 Audit of mental health assessments (n = 43)

	Satisfactorily recorded items	Percentage satisfactory out of relevant denominator (not always 43)
History		
Timing of onset	40	93
Symptomatic description	41	95
Drug history	31	72
Occupation		
Qualitative workload	20	49
Quantitative workload	14	34
Past history	41	95
Possible substance misuse	20	51
Examination		
Affect (mood)	23	56
Diagnosis/conclusions		
Nature of condition	41	95
Causative factors	35	81
Advice/action		
Work fitness	42	98
Stress reduction measures	33	83

This audit suggested a generally satisfactory management of workers many of whom had presented themselves. It led to debate on the need to pursue tactfully the possibility of substance abuse, and also to make explicit records on the subject's mood in case either of these warranted more active intervention. It permitted a consensus to be reached on the need for more formal quantitative evaluation of occupational stress and stressors in that workforce.

Routinely collecting information, such as sickness absence data and other 'health outcome' data, has been advocated as a means of evaluating OHS or occupational health performance in the workplace. However, such 'data' should be treated very cautiously, since the diagnoses attributed to certified ill-health are subject to considerable error and bias.

Moreover, it is well known that the extent of absence attributed to sickness – although often including a substantial proportion of work-related ill-health – may correlate very poorly with it. Other outcomes may be considered, such as premature ill-health retirements. In this context, it may be worthwhile to audit retirement decisions or recommendations against a set of valid criteria. This would be a very useful exercise in itself, since if inconsistent practice is revealed steps can be taken to remedy this through education or policy changes. If, on the other hand, ill-health retirement recommendations are found to be generally valid, then their frequency – classified by ill-health category – could be a useful prospective audit tool for the organization as a whole.

Closing the audit loop

An audit is of little practical value unless the 'loop' is closed. In other words, after observed practice has been compared with the standard, reasons for deviation from the standard must be debated, remedial steps designed and measures implemented. Further audit of the new practice against the standard is important to demonstrate improvement. Quantitative assessment methods can indicate not only what is wrong, but can also suggest why – and hence lead to specific remedies (see Boxes 5.2 and 5.6–5.9 for examples).

Results of audits should be discussed in a non-confrontational manner with all concerned, bearing in mind that even one set of results of a quantitative evaluation can allow a range of different interpretations and actions. Throughout all of this, an 'audit trail' must be pursued, so that it is clear as to what decision has been taken, why, by whom and when that decision is due for review.

All details as to size, location and identification of the sampling frame, sampling ratio, abstraction of data and analysis, must be accurately kept, and made available for scrutiny. Further, in seeking to improve quality, the 'law of diminishing returns' should be borne in mind. There comes a point when it is more productive to seek improvements in a hitherto uncharted area than to invest even more resources in converting a well-trodden and viable path into a perfect highway.

One should also consider that quantitative methods themselves need to be subject to change and re-evaluation so that they can improve by a process of iteration (see Box 5.10).

Box 5.10 Reproducibility of the audit tools

An external audit of occupational health consultations originally conducted by a specialist occupational physician was repeated (blind) by a second external auditor on a set of 68 consultations. Kappa coefficients (K) (a better method of determining inter-observer reproducibility than simply percentage agreement) were calculated for the items in the audit.

- An almost perfect strength of agreement was only found for the basic identifying information such as classification of occupational category ($K = 0.91$).
- Substantial agreement was found for items such as the underlying ($K = 0.77$), the primary clinical problem ($K=0.78$) and whether there had been communication with the General Practitioner following sickness absence consultation ($K = 0.64$).

- Moderate agreement was found for items such as the presence of a follow-up plan for the employee ($K = 0.46$) and recorded communication with the employer ($K = 0.58$).
- Fair agreement was found between the auditors' conclusions on the extent to which an adequate physical examination had been conducted ($K = 0.36$), on whether a specific diagnosis had been reached ($K = 0.39$), or on the extent to which the consultations had made a judgement on the likely date of return to work following sickness absence ($K = 0.33$).
- However only slight or poor agreement was found between the auditors on many items such as the extent to which the audited consultations reached conclusions on whether work could be affecting the employee's health ($K = 0.16$), on residual disability or level of fitness ($K = 0.09$), on likely duration of any residual disability ($K = 0.09$) or provided advice on rehabilitation ($K = 0.16$).

These data suggest either that the audit criteria or supporting guidelines need to be improved, or that the observers need more consistent training. One can conclude that the degree of agreement between different observers, the detail of definition of audit criteria, and the extent of training of auditors have to be very carefully considered when using audit tools. If significant divergence between auditors persists this can be a useful basis for improving the tools and for education. However, where quantitative methods are to be used for the purposes of ranking quality then a high degree of inter-observer agreement and hence reproducibility is necessary.

Concluding remarks

Audit is one of many tools for achieving quality in OHS. If all of these tools were pursued to the extent to which they are individually advocated, a large amount of resources would need to be invested. If these show a limited return, serious inefficiency could arise. Moreover, if an inappropriate choice of standards, or of methods is made, false conclusions may be drawn about an OHS organization, and ineffective – or even counter-productive – changes implemented. The ideal way of proceeding is to devise and implement the correct system and to apply appropriate competencies 'first time'.

Scientific research must be conducted to determine appropriate standards, and also to understand the complex relationships between process and outcome. The pressure for quality improvement, and the advent of third-party audits may help in some circumstances. However, if such pressure results in arbitrary quality standards or in auditing what can be audited rather than what should, unwarranted self-satisfaction may be generated. The occupational health literature shows encouraging signs of evidence-based consensus in a number of areas, and demonstrates various audit and evaluation initiatives. Quantitative methods have to be accompanied by the oldest of qualitative methods – 'listening', where all concerned are partners. Against such a background, audit and quantitative evaluation are likely to bear fruit by way of an improvement in the effectiveness and efficiency of services, and the achievement of a universally recognized high level of practice.

Acknowledgements

Part of the work forming the background to this chapter was funded by a research fellowship from the Faculty of Occupational Medicine of the Royal College of Physicians of London. The cooperation and support of health boards, and other workplaces in Scotland during pilot work on auditing OHS, are also gratefully acknowledged. Several occupational health professionals have contributed to the work described here, including M. Gaffney, V. Riddle, A. Seaton, and I. Symington.

References

Agius, R.M. (1995) Occupational asthma and rhinitis. Part III −Health surveillance and secondary prevention. *Occup. Hlth Rev.*, May/June., pp. 28–31.

Agius, R.M., Lee, R.J., Murdoch, R.M., Symington, I.S., Riddle, H.F.V. and Seaton, A. (1993) Occupational physicians and their work: prospects for audit. *Occup. Med.*, **43**, 159–63.

Agius, R.M., Lee, R.J., Symington, I.S., Riddle, H.F.V. and Seaton, A. (1994) An audit of occupational medicine consultation records. *Occup. Med.*, **44**, 151–7.

Agius, R.M., Seaton, A. and Lee, R.J.(1995) Audit of sickness absence and fitness-for-work referrals. *Occup. Med.* 1995; **45**, 125–30.

Crombie, I.K. and Davies, H.T.O (1998) Beyond health outcomes: the advantages of measuring process. *J. Evalu. Clin. Pract.*, **4**, 31–8.

Husman, K. (1993) Principles and pitfalls in health services research in occupational health systems. *Occup. Med.*, **43** (Suppl 1), S10–S14.

MacDonald, E.B. (ed.), Agius, R.M., McCloy, E.C., McCulloch, W.J.M., Miller, D.M., Paterson, J.C. and Whitaker, S. (1995) *Quality and Audit in Occupational Health*. London: Faculty of Occupational Medicine of the Royal College of Physicians of London.

Seaton, A., Agius, R., McCloy, E. and D'Auria, D. (1994) *Practical Occupational Medicine*. Appendix 5: *Audit in Occupational Medicine*. London: Edward Arnold, pp. 259–264.

van der Weide, W.E., Verbeek, J.H.A.M., van Dijk, F.J.H. and Doef, J. (1997) An audit of occupational health care for employees with low-back pain. *Occup. Med.*, **47**, 294–300.

van der Weide, W.E., Verbeek, J.H.A.M., van Dijk, F.J.H. and Hulshof, C.T.J (1998) Development and evaluation of a quality assessment instrument for occupational physicians. *Occup. Environ. Med.*, **55**, 375–82.

Westerholm, P. (1995) Measurement of outcome. In: *Epidemiology of Work Related Diseases* (C. McDonald, ed.). London: BMJ Publishing Group, pp. 387–412.

Whitaker, S. and Aw, T-C. (1995) Audit of pre-employment assessments by occupational health departments in the National Health Service. *Occup. Med.*, **45**:75–80.

6

Major evaluation models pertinent to OHS practice

Ewa Menckel

The theory and practice of evaluation has developed with great rapidity over the past two decades. Originally introduced in the educational arena, it has made inroads in a wide range of fields (including public health, and more specifically occupational health). Broadly speaking, evaluations are either summative (performed retrospectively to assess a project outcome) or formative (designed to impact on a project in progress). On the basis of the concepts of consensus and freedom of choice, House (1978) developed a taxonomy of eight evaluation models. These range, according to their audiences and main topics addressed, from what he calls Systems Analysis to Transaction. Each of these is described, and their features related to the practical examples of OHS evaluation described in the latter section of this book.

Evaluation models and OHS work

Over the past 20 years, a wide variety of frameworks, models and methods for evaluation work has been created. The field of evaluation has been enriched by contributions from many disciplines and professional activities, a number of which have left a profound imprint. Many evaluators have come from the field of education. Concepts such as summative and formative evaluation (Weiss, 1972) and goal-free evaluation (Scriven, 1975) have been developed and put into practice (see also Chapter 2). But what do these concepts and approaches stand for? How can they be compared and implemented? What types of issues do they strive to address? Are any of them really applicable to the evaluation of occupational health services (OHS) practice? Are the 'typical questions' to which they give rise relevant in this arena?

The purpose of this chapter is to highlight some assumptions underlying evaluation and to offer a basis for discussing which of different models or methods should/can be chosen to evaluate OHS work. The chapter is a revised version of part of an earlier report on models and methods that OHS might employ in evaluation work (Menckel, 1993).

In this first section of this book – the more theory-oriented section – a number of general principles of and models for evaluation are presented.

One of the ways in which evaluation models can be distinguished is according to whether they are summative or formative. The distinction illustrates how evaluations can differ with regard to goals, time of initiation and focus. In this chapter, however, a wider range of evaluation models and differences between them are presented. The chapter can also be seen as an introduction to Part 2 – the more practically oriented part – of the book, as the various kinds of evaluation models presented will be reflected in the different case studies of OHS work it provides.

The account is based on House's (1978) elaborate and systematic analysis of the idea of evaluation and the specific characteristics of the various models he identifies. His taxonomy of major evaluation models is one of the most frequently referred to and one of the few attempts to provide an analytical framework to organize the multidisciplinary nature of evaluation (Rootman *et al.*, 1997). As the chapter concerns models and methods, we start by offering definitions of model and method in this context:

- a **model** is a simplified picture of reality, a graphic cognitive schema for describing an abstract, complex phenomenon;
- a **method** is a systematic means for gathering and processing facts, a pre-scheduled manner of proceeding in order to achieve certain results.

The importance of clarity and consensus with regard to the aim of an evaluation has already been pointed to (Chapter 2). Consensus (or lack of consensus) can be a guiding principle in choice of evaluation model. But lack of consensus need not mean a lack of agreement over what is to be evaluated or elucidated; rather, it is over what outcomes follow from a measure taken, and how these are to be evaluated that disagreements arise. The differences may be many and varied. Highlighting them serves to elucidate varying conceptions of the nature of the activity at hand.

Assumptions underlying evaluation models

House argues that all evaluation models have their origin in the philosophy of liberalism. In his view, liberalism itself arose from an attempt to rationalize and give legitimacy to market society on the basis of the principle of **freedom of choice.** Freedom of choice is also a fundamental feature of the evaluation models, although there can be disagreement over which and whose choices are encompassed by them. A second fundamental feature of liberalism, relevant to the evaluation models identified by House, is the primacy of **the psychology of the individual,** i.e. the individual has an existence prior to that of society although he/she is gradually incorporated into it. A further idea, to be found in liberalism and of relevance to the models, is **empiricism**, which in its extreme form amounts to the claim that everything can be derived from observation. All evaluation models have what House calls an 'empiricist flavour'.

The evaluation models also assume a market in ideas, in the sense that people are free to adopt whatever views they wish. Thus, evaluation in a totalitarian state is regarded as an impossibility. It is competition between ideas which promotes the truth. The knowledge acquired by human beings makes them happier and better as human beings. Thus, a concept that is fundamental to evaluation is freedom of choice; without freedom of choice there is no evaluation – for what is the point of evaluation if no choice can be made?

In all House's eight evaluation models there is a striving to achieve a state that is 'good'. The top four models (see Table 6.1) are all 'utilitarian', i.e. the greatest possible happiness in society is the superordinate goal. In these models there is an attempt to achieve a universally accepted judgement on what is perceived to be of general social benefit – sometimes in terms of a small number of criteria (as, for example, in the Systems Analysis model), sometimes using a large number (as in the Goal Free model). The four models at the bottom focus more on utility for the individual, and have what House describes as a 'subjectivist' emphasis. Social/societal utility has been replaced by personal understanding, diversity and the acceptance of divergent points of view.

The 'social utility' models make use of accepted, explicit methodologies, and objective, usually quantitative and reproducible, methods and measures. Knowledge is explicit, clear and explanatory. By contrast, in the other models, it is implicit, tacit and with a focus on understanding. In the latter cases, more subjective and qualitative methods can be employed.

A review of evaluation models

Table 6.1 shows – in simplified form – House's taxonomy of eight major evaluation models, which he derived from a review of a large number of classifications and descriptions of different types of evaluations. In his original work he used the following critical dimensions to compare and classify the models: the audience to whom the evaluation is addressed, on what the model 'assumes consensus', methodology, the ultimate outcome expected and the typical questions addressed. Table 6.1 shows 'Major audiences' and the 'Major topics addressed'.

Table 6.1 *A taxonomy of major evaluation models (adapted from House, 1978)*

Model	Major audiences	Main topic addressed
Systems Analysis	Economists, managers	Overall expected effects
Behavioural Objectives	Managers, psychologists	Specific, objective effects/performances
Decision-making	Decision-makers, esp. administrators	Stepwise (partial) effects
Goal Free	Consumers	All and any effects
Art Criticism	Connoisseurs, consumers	Critical approval
Accreditation	Teachers, public	Professional rating
Adversary	Jury	Conflict resolution
Transaction	Clients, practitioners	Understanding of the learning process

In the taxonomy above the models are systematically related to each other. In general, the further one descends the 'Major audiences' column in Table 6.1, the more democratic, or less élitist, the model becomes. The three models highest up in the column assume that there is consensus on which result criteria are to be employed in the evaluation, a consensus that is usually based on the possibility of a rather small number of persons with major decision-making capacity reaching agreement. In the Goal Free model consensus has also been achieved in that there is agreement over the existence of a number of further criteria, although it has not been possible to lay these down in advance. The other four models are more pluralist by nature. But even in these, there is agreement over how the evaluator is to be appointed, and which procedures are needed to carry out the evaluation.

Also, the models are so arranged that the further one descends the columns, the greater is the number of people with which the evaluation is concerned; more persons become involved and participate. Note that these are simplifications; the actual orders are more complicated.

There follows below a description of each of the eight models, with illustrations of how they are reflected in the different examples/cases of evaluation of OHS work provided in the second part of this book. House himself provides a list of the 'typical questions' raised by each kind of evaluation. We refer to some of these, and add others that may be more pertinent in an OHS context.

The Systems Analysis model

This model assumes consensus on overall goals and on various cause–effect relations. It further presupposes that there are some (few) quantifiable measures to which the programme, project or any other major activity to be evaluated is related. The information gathered is usually wide-ranging by nature and the analysis is based on a variety of statistical/mathematical methods, such as correlation or cost–benefit appraisal. An evaluation following this model should provide illumination with regard to some form of specific, overall and ultimate effect.

The evaluation is carried out for authorities, economists, corporate executives and organizations. Also, it is these persons who determine which measures are to be used, and when and how the evaluation is to be carried out.

The aim of an application of the model is to provide a superordinate valuation of an entire body of activities. It can, for example, be employed to assess whether an operation has achieved its goals or been of 'social' utility. It can also be used to compare different programmes or major projects so as to judge which of them is best, cheapest or the most efficient. It is always summative by nature and is initiated after an operation has been completed or after it has been in progress for a specific period of time.

With regard to the work of OHS, this model can, for example, be used to assess overall operations in relation to other activities on the basis of a specific measure, e.g. cost effectiveness.

Typical questions
- Are the expected effects achieved?
- Can the effects be achieved more economically?
- What are the most *efficient* programmes?
- What conditions are most favourable for achieving ...?

OHS-related questions
- Have OHS achieved the goals stipulated by law and agreement?
- Has the work of OHS led to a better work environment?
- Can a good work environment be achieved more economically than via OHS?
- Can OHS contribute to a reduction in occupational diseases/injuries?
- What type of OHS care gives the best results?

An example of a Systems Analysis approach is offered by the Japanese case. In this evaluation study, the characteristics of OHS in Japan were compared to international standards using a conceptual framework (structure, process and outcome) and five documents (three domestic and two international). The purpose was to clarify the problems of current Japanese OHS from an international perspective. Although the evaluation was based largely on structural and process-oriented measures, the aim was to assess an entire body of activities – so as to shed light upon which parts of Japanese OHS could be improved and how such improvement could be achieved. In this sense, the intention of the evaluation and the evaluation procedure can be seen as following a Systems Analysis model.

A further example of analysis according to the Systems Analysis model lies in the work conducted by the Norwegian team. The evaluators were commissioned by the government to assess the present function of OHS in Norway and give answers to questions such as: 'To what extent do enterprises use OHS to perform the tasks stipulated in the Work Environment Law?', and 'Do the activities/actions performed by OHS lead to concrete results/effects in enterprises?' The team developed a conceptual model for their evaluation based on interaction between an enterprise and its related OHS. They used both quantitative methods (at national level) and qualitative techniques (case studies). Accordingly, the evaluation can be regarded as following both a Systems Analysis and Transaction model (see below).

The Behavioural Objectives model

A programme or an operation's goal is formulated in terms of performances or products. The model was used originally in schools to measure the results and performances achieved by pupils and teachers. It was assumed that these could be stipulated in specific, objective measures. Here too, it is persons in authority, administrators and professionals (such as directors of studies, doctors and psychologists) who determine the criteria and implement the evaluation. The model assumes consensus on these criteria, on which objectives are to be measured and evaluated. School performance, for example, is measured by grades, examinations, tests etc.

This evaluation model is probably the most commonly used, and is in many respects the easiest to apply. It assumes consensus on which effects are to be measured, and also which outcomes are related to which specific inputs or efforts made. The outcomes of a particular effort (a performance) can then be more easily measured and evaluated.

Even in the OHS arena, this model may be the simplest to utilize – largely because it is designed to measure and evaluate the outcome of a specific action taken. Usually, OHS personnel can themselves become involved in implementation.

Typical questions
• Has the objective been achieved?
• Has the programme increased knowledge?
• Does a certain activity have the expected outcome?

OHS-related questions
• Have OHS staff achieved their specific goals/objectives?
• Have company visits led to proposals for measures?
• Have back exercises led to improved physical fitness?
• Have rehabilitation activities led to shorter periods of sick leave?

The outcome-based evaluation of OHS in the USA provides an example of the application of the Behavioural Objectives model. Specific outcomes of a comprehensive occupational health and safety programme in a delimited region were evaluated. The authors point to the importance of outcome evaluation, based on relevant measures, as means of pointing OHS in new directions for improvement.

A further example of the application of a Behavioural Objectives model lies in the Swedish case of process-oriented evaluation of OHS rehabilitation work. The aim of this project was to describe, monitor and analyse the different activities of OHS personnel in order to see whether they had improved their contacts with other actors in the rehabilitation process (e.g. with personnel at rehabilitation institutions and the workplaces involved). These activities could be seen as reflecting a form of Behavioural Objectives model, but also as involving a Transaction model (see below) in that they focused on understanding of the learning process and giving OHS staff an opportunity to see solutions and initiate changes.

The Decision-Making model

As with the Systems Analysis and Behavioural Objectives models, the aim of this approach is to supply managerial staff with information. Its focus is on giving persons in responsible positions a basis on which they can evaluate and reach decisions on the continuing operation of a programme or project.

What distinguishes this evaluation model from the two described above is that the evaluations are structured through decisions taken as the operation develops. The evaluator's task is to acquire information at each stage and relay this to decision-makers. The information refers to different steps in operations, different parts of a programme (or a set of measures) and concerns what each part has resulted in.

Methods employed include 'surveys, questionnaires, interviews' and analysis of the 'natural variation' in operations. Quality control is a term that often comes up in this context.

The model can be employed in the evaluation work of OHS in order to supply different managers with information on activities, their different parts, what has led to what, and what has worked well/less well on an ongoing basis.

Typical questions
• Is the programme effective?
• What parts are effective?
• How effective is the work put in at each phase?

OHS-related questions
• Have planned training measures been implemented?
• Have these increased knowledge, e.g. on hazards at work?
• Has this in turn contributed to safer working methods?
• Which parts of workplace investigations are effective?
• Is the rehabilitation programme in the workplace being implemented?
• Which parts of the programme have proved to have which effects (economic, social, production-related)?

The example from the Canadian Province of Quebec has elements of Decision-Making evaluation as it is aimed at decision-makers on different levels. The evaluation is based on an extensive statistical implementation analysis of a public occupational health programme.

A second example is the occupational health audit programme described in the UK case.

The Goal Free model

This model is, at one and the same time, both the easiest and most difficult to use – easiest in that it assumes the consensus that relevant criteria and outcomes can emerge in the course of an evaluation (it is important to take account of these); the difficulty may come in gaining a hearing for the results of such evaluations among, for example, decision-makers and owners.

The model caused rather a storm when it was first employed in the mid-1970s in the USA. This was because it is not based on 'prespecified objectives' in its analysis of activities or the implementation and results of a programme. Many regarded it as controversial.

The aim of the model is to illuminate a programme from as many different angles as possible. This means being alert and sensitive to different kinds of effects and results, even those which are believed initially not be of any significance. Different measures and analyses must then be assessed and combined into a kind of general summative judgement. The procedure can be likened to the work conducted in an association or group, where the views of all the different persons involved have to find expression. The 'ultimate result' is a general judgement on 'better' and 'best', in which is included an evaluation of best choice and social utility.

This model provides scope for reducing the weight of preconceived opinions in an evaluation. By consciously searching for effects other than those envisaged by managers or others, the evaluator can highlight many interesting aspects of an operation or efforts made. The opinions of the different persons involved can find expression. Relatively simple quantitative and qualitative methods can be employed, alongside logical analysis, bias control, observations, inspection of case-books etc.

The Goal Free model can be hard to employ in OHS work, since it is a comprehensive approach and can generate extensive and diffuse information for which it is difficult to obtain an overview. However, it may reveal unintended outcomes to which the company/client can give greater priority than those initially addressed by the evaluation.

Typical questions
• What are *all* the effects?'
• Are there other effects which have not found expression?
• What effects do different persons perceive there to be?

OHS-related questions
• To what effects do OHS clients/companies give priority?
• What are the opinions of OHS clients on training measures?
• What are the consequences for OHS personnel?

The Goal Free model in its pure form has such special characteristics that it is hard to find examples of it among the cases in the second section of this book. However, several of the evaluations described have components that demonstrate sensitivity to unintended effects which have surfaced in the course of the work. These have then been evaluated and taken account of in decision-making.

They may concern clients' opinions, effects within a company that could not have been foreseen, or particular efforts which have pushed evaluation work forwards despite not being initially included in the evaluation. Examples are available in the two Swedish evaluation cases, and also in the Norwegian case. In all three, personal interviews or group interviews were used to highlight, discuss and assess different activities and measures taken by OHS staff or others in the course of the ongoing evaluation work.

The Art Criticism model

This model has been developed from the tradition of art and literary criticism, where various documents and sources are scrutinized to assess a piece of work, a course of events or an effort made. In this tradition a number of standards and norms have been developed, which function as the basis on which a critical assessment is made.

The model aims at improving operations or a programme by utilizing the knowledge that professional evaluators ('critics') can offer. Long experience and training has put them in possession of principles and norms and developed them into specialized judges. A variety of methods of critical analysis are employed in evaluation.

OHS activities can, for example, be assessed from a number of critical perspectives – historical, political, financial, or in terms of implications for the labour market or health. The same applies to individual efforts and actions. The evaluation can point to various critical points or events that may be of significance for continued operations.

Typical questions
• Would a critic approve this programme?
• What key points/events can be identified?
• Would a critic be able to improve . . .?

OHS-related questions
• How would an educational specialist rate OHS training activities?
• Have OHS the 'right' formula for reviewing . . .?

An example might be an outside evaluator, researcher or research team being allotted the task of assessing OHS operations (either as a whole or in part). This happened in the Norwegian case and the UK case. Another might be the appointment of a panel to review activities in some specific aspect.

Cases of panels reviewing the OHS work were evident in some of our examples. The evaluation of OHS in the Mexican Institute of Social Security is based on a strategic programme for occupational health that encompasses norms, research, information, meetings, education and training. These elements jointly form a model that operates at different levels in the organization. Support is then provided by a tripartite committee, which evaluates/assesses OHS activities and their effects on the health of the working population.

The Accreditation model

In this model accreditation (i.e. authorization) is given to an activity, person or product on the basis of pre-set criteria. Examples of such accreditation in everyday life include the authority to judge cars to be roadsafe (vehicle testing), the practice of certain professions (e.g. author-ized accountancy), the setting-up of certain product standards (e.g. for electrical appliances). The evaluation involves approving (or not approv-ing) a product, performance or activity on the basis of certain, specific professional expertise. Usually, the professional who is to carry out the rating is appointed by the government or other authority.

The methods employed stem from decisions founded on major re-views, the discussions of panels of experts or specific 'self studies'. They are usually well documented, but their origins and application will be largely a matter of intuitive professional judgement based on many years' experience.

Typical questions
- How would professionals rate this programme?'
- Is the activity practised by competent personnel?
- Is the activity practised in accordance with established criteria?

OHS-related questions
- Is OHS work mainly preventive by nature?
- Does OHS have medical, technical and psychosocial expertise?
- Have staff gone through adequate OHS training?

An example of an evaluation with Accreditation elements is the UK case. Questionnaires and also peer review were utilized in a national audit of pre-employment assessments as part of a professional rating procedure. Professional ratings also come up in the German example. In many of the cases, standard documents (such as ISO-9000) have been used to evaluate OHS work.

The Adversary model

Many have made use of quasi-legal procedures to examine a programme or to bring to light its advantages and disadvantages. This model, the Adversary model, enables a systematic account of the views and assessments of contesting parties to be presented. The evaluation often takes the form of a trial by jury, where the jury has complete freedom to employ a multiplicity of diverse criteria in an intuitive manner. The adversaries have the right to present any type of evidence they consider relevant, in whatever form. The different parties may have widely divergent views and set quite different standards for a programme's goal achievement.

The model is designed to resolve a conflict by highlighting and assessing arguments for and against a programme or activity. Quasi-legal procedures are employed.

Typical questions
- What are the arguments for and against the programme?
- How can a conflict be resolved?
- How can the views of the different parties be balanced and judged?

OHS-related questions
- How do the client and OHS each look at occupational health care?
- Should OHS continue with certain types of health check-ups?
- What do OHS and the client each want from OHS?

This evaluation model seems to have its greatest utility in relation to the marketing of OHS activities and the drawing-up of contracts between OHS and their clients. If the ideas underlying this model are employed, then the evaluation that OHS and their client should jointly conduct after the completion of an OHS performance can be facilitated.

There is no clear-cut example of the application of an Adversary evaluation model among the cases described in Part 2. There is, however, a hint of an adversarial approach in the way the Norwegian Ministry of

Local Government and Labour highlighted the customers of OHS and their opinions. One aim was to find out whether OHS could function as an instrument for improvements pursuant to the Work Environment Act of 1977. This may be seen as a form of highlighting and assessing arguments for and against various parts of OHS work. The evaluation of Japanese OHS might also be seen as having an adversarial element.

The Transaction model

Finally we come to the Transaction model. In this a multiplicity of diverse criteria are introduced, so that the different people involved may present their opinions and make their own judgements. By illuminating how these persons are affected and how they perceive the results of the influences on them, understanding is created over, for example, how learning takes place, and how a programme has been received and implemented. This understanding is based on the perspectives of those involved.

Case studies, interviews and observations are all employed in this context. The data are assessed by both the evaluator and the participants.

Typical questions
• What does the programme look like to different people?
• How have different people acted/been affected?
• What has been the nature of the interaction between people?

OHS-related questions
• How have OHS personnel been affected by the activity?
• How has the relationship between OHS and client been affected?

There is a sense in which it is both difficult and easy to find examples of this evaluation model – difficult in that it is seldom applied in pure form (for it requires a lot of time, personnel and other resources in order to obtain comprehensive coverage); easy in that there are elements of the model in so many evaluations that are carried out in practice.

One of the Swedish cases – concerned with rehabilitation of work-related musculoskeletal disorders – might be said to follow the Transaction model. The evaluators implemented a problem-based learning procedure to involve all participants in rehabilitation development and to include psychosocial resources in the rehabilitation process.

Concluding remarks

Of the eight models in House's classification, the Behavioural Objectives model (what might be called a 'performance' approach) is the most widely employed. It is designed to shed light on a specific outcome, on the basis of such questions as 'Have objectives been achieved?', or 'Have intended effects been demonstrated?'. It presupposes a specifically demarcated, measurable performance, which is to be evaluated and followed up, in a context where the different parties involved can reach agreement on what is to be evaluated. Probably it is the simplest model to start with when embarking on the evaluation of specific activities or measures taken by OHS.

Some of the other models, such as the Systems Analysis and Transaction models, require greater, more radical efforts. A model that can provide inspiration is the Goal Free model, where a search is made for what is not known, and which is open to effects and consequences that cannot be foreseen.

> 'Finally, we evaluate the result. The experience makes us wiser, and maybe we are given new ideas which we can test the next time. In this process we form the different elements into a meaningful whole. Thought and action go together.'(*Work for Change.* The Swedish Work Environment Fund's OHS Programme, 1991)

References

House, E.R. (1978) Assumptions underlying evaluation models. *Educ. Researcher*, 7, 7–12.

Menckel, E. (1993) *Evaluating and Promoting Change in Occupational Health Services. Models and Applications.* The Swedish Work Environment Fund.

Rootman, I., Goodstadt, M., Potvin, L. and Springett, J. (1977) *Toward a Framework for Health Promotion Evaluation.* WHO Regional Office for Europe, Copenhagen.

Scriven, M. (1975) The methodology of evaluation. From Popham WJ In: *Educational Evaluation* (W.J. Popham, ed.). Englewood Cliffs, NJ: Prentice–Hall.

Weiss, C.H. (1972) *Evaluation Research. Methods for Assessing Programme Effectiveness.* (Methods of Social Science Series.) Englewood Cliffs, NJ: Prentice–Hall.

Part 2
EVALUATION IN PRACTICE

7

OHS evaluation – principles, approaches and methods

Peter Westerholm and Ewa Menckel

This chapter deals with general principles to bear in mind when approaching an occupational health services (OHS) unit or programme/project with the intention to evaluate. Basic approaches to planning and conducting an evaluation are considered, starting with definitions of important concepts. Motives and objectives of evaluation, and the related questions of who carries out an evaluation, and what its object should be are also dealt with. Aspects of data collection are only touched upon, but their dependence on end-objectives is emphasized. Formative and summative evaluations are explained, and the stakeholder concept as a tenet of social-programme evaluation highlighted. Finally, there is a short discussion of quantitative and qualitative methods.

The concept of evaluation has to be defined at the very outset. From this follows the basic questions of why?, what?, when?, and for whom? to evaluate. Following examination of these questions, it is time to address the issue of method – the question of how? There is a very close relationship between objectives of a programme/project, and the appropriate procedure and methods for its evaluation, and this will have a bearing on the planning of an evaluation.

A few important terms

We start with a few key expressions:

- **Evaluator:** a person doing an evaluation.
- **The evaluated:** the item (programme/project/activity) or intervention which is evaluated – the subject of the evaluation.
- **Target:** the part or whole of the (working) population that the evaluated aims to affect (NB *not* the target of the evaluation).
- **Sponsor:** the person who initiates or pays for the evaluation.
- **User:** the person who makes use of or acts on the evaluation.

> ## Reminder
>
> Evaluations differ according to:
>
> - **Object** of evaluation (priorities, preventive or remedial actions, interventions, surveillance programmes etc.).
> - **Target group** of evaluation (professional categories, key persons in client enterprises, OHS unit staff etc.).
> - **Purpose** of evaluation (to decide whether programme works, improvement of performance, ascertainment of return on invested funding).
> - **User** of evaluation (OHS professionals, managers, enterprises, trade unions, external bodies).
> - **Design** of evaluation (descriptive, analytic).
> - **Methods** used in evaluation (quantitative, qualitative, direct observations, measurements).

A definition of evaluation

Evaluation is attributing value to the evaluated by gathering reliable and valid information about it in a systematic way and by making comparisons, for the purpose of making more informed decisions or understanding causal mechanisms or general principles (Øvretveit, 1998).

Some points in this definition deserve special emphasis.

The evaluated – this denotes the thing or object whose value is to be assessed. It may include health treatments, interventions, occupational health practices such as health surveillance, risk assessments, or changes in organizations or work processes with health or risk implications.

Attributing value – this is a central aspect. Valuation means that value criteria are to be applied. The questions are then – Whose value criteria? Are there norms or standards? Professional criteria? Users' criteria? Management criteria? It is important for the evaluator to be aware that these different sets of values may lead to differing expectations concerning the results of an evaluation and the inferences to be drawn from it.

Making comparisons – value is most often assessed on the basis of comparison. This, in fact, is the essence of quality valuation. Quality – in terms of quality-standard systems nomenclature – is the capacity of a product or service to satisfy specified requirements or expectations. This means that a comparison is made between what is observed and what has been expected. The observations made during an evaluation may also be compared with norms or standard documents. Recommendations are then given in guidelines or codes of practice, or in relation to observations made at a similar health service unit selected as a basis for reference. Another type of comparison – 'before-and-after' – is made on one and the same evaluation object with a view to assessing the impact of an action taken.

Better informed decisions – the purpose of an evaluation is to add to information already available by highlighting aspects conducive to awareness and improvement of performance. This applies to the various stakeholders involved among OHS professionals, managers, users of OHS, and many others.

The decision-making aspect is particularly important. It deals with the end-objective of an evaluation (NB *not* the end-objective of what is being evaluated). It is essential to specify what type of decision is envisaged, and for what an evaluation is to be used. Is it to see whether the evaluated service has the effects that were assumed or hypothesized when it started? This reflects the control function of the evaluation. Or is the question rather 'Why have no effects resulted from this programme of the OHS and what can be done to improve it?' This implies an evaluation with an objective to promote or improve a process or service activity.

What can evaluations do?

An evaluation does not implement change. Rather, it produces an improved basis for decision-making, with a view to acting on observations made. The two following points can be made about an ideal evaluation:

- An evaluation helps those concerned in attributing value to what is being evaluated.
- An evaluation has a clear objective in itself. It may aim at a description of what is being evaluated or an explanation of what is observed in a programme or service – usually with a view to improvement (see our discussion of evaluation design below).

Why evaluate?

This question basically focuses on the need to specify the occasion on which OHS programmes, projects or practices should be evaluated. Important reasons include:

- to assess the effectiveness/impact of a programme or action;
- to explain or explore opportunities to improve effectiveness and efficiency;
- to reappraise priorities and uses of resources;
- to assess the needs and demands of client groups;
- to assess the efficiency (cost/benefit) of programmes;
- to improve knowledge and the decision-making base of management and occupational health professionals;
- to respond to external pressures.

Evaluations may be requested by important stakeholder categories, such as governmental agencies, customer groups and others.

There is an increasing awareness among occupational health practitioners and professionals of the importance of understanding the principles of evaluation. Such understanding generates capacity to:

- understand and grasp information in an evaluation report, and to adapt it to one's own organization and OHS unit;

- apply evaluation principles in one's own work, and review the work organization and performance of one's own unit.

Who evaluates?

This is an important question, which should be addressed at an early stage. It determines – and is also determined by – the arena chosen and the evaluation's audience and results. There are basically three levels:

- **Self-evaluation**. This is done by OHS practitioners or OHS units themselves with the aim of improving their own performance and quality. Such an evaluation is usually carried out in an internal arena, e.g. the OHS unit involved.
- **Internal evaluation**. This is carried out within an organization by specially designated persons. It might, for example, target a company's own OHS unit. In such a case, the arena of evaluation is the company.
- **External evaluation**. This is conducted by evaluators external to the company or service involved. It may be done on behalf of a customer organization – a practice sometimes referred to as second-party evaluation, or by an independent body (such as a certified quality-standard assessing organization) – referred to as a third party evaluation. One particular type of external evaluation is that carried out by a public health agency. This may imply that the arena of evaluation is 'public'.

Common questions for evaluators

A good practical rule of thumb in planning evaluations is to frame the questions to be addressed at an early stage. A good evaluation is always capable of answering questions defined at the outset. Common questions are:

- Does the occupational health programme or service item work? Is it effective in an ideal situation only or in most ordinary contexts? Does it work only on certain conditions?
- What do we mean by good OHS performance?
- Why does the programme/service item work, or not work?
- What are its effects, including unintended and long-term consequences of the programme?
- How durable are its effects?
- What were the costs?
- Was it cost-effective in comparison with some other way of doing it?
- What did we learn from it in terms of our own productivity, professional competence and organization?
- What do our customers think about it?
- What is the utility value of the services provided by the OHS organization? Is it conducive to preventive action, improvement of work conditions or quality of life at work?
- What do occupational health professionals think about it?
- How can it be improved?

- Does it meet established official or non-official standards, and is it consistent with current regulations?
- Should it be stopped or should it be allowed to continue?

Basic principles

Evaluations are commonly carried out to assess an organization, a service commodity, or an action or intervention undertaken with a view to bring about a change.

In planning an evaluation, one of the first essential steps is to analyse the process or function to be evaluated. This is done with a view to familiarizing ourselves with it and getting to know how it works. This also applies to individual service items provided by OHS, such as pre-employment medical examinations, workplace visits and workplace-based alcohol/drug abuse prevention programmes.

Many factors may contribute to and significantly influence the workings and performances of an OHS organization. Examples of such factors are health and safety regulations, the organizational culture of the service unit, physical and psychological workplace characteristics, work conditions in companies served, characteristics of populations served, and the competencies and skills of the professional and other staff at the OHS unit concerned. The occupational health policies and management of customer enterprises, and the policies and task conceptions of OHS themselves are other important factors. Such contextual factors need to be taken into account when evaluating OHS organizations and programmes.

The four basic steps in an evaluation

Evaluation is an assessment, and should be seen as a project. In leading an evaluation project some basic elements of the undertaking should be clarified and kept in mind. These are:

- the objectives and scope of the evaluation;
- the resources necessary to carry out the evaluation;
- for whom the evaluation is carried out and on what contractual terms;
- to whom the evaluator is expected to report the evaluation findings.

If the evaluation is undertaken with a view to issuing a certificate this should be set out clearly in the evaluation agreement. In general, such formal agreements should include a clear description of expectations and an unambiguous account of the tasks to be carried out.

A simple rule of thumb in planning an evaluation procedure is to apply a structured, methodical approach. The following general instructions may be used as a basis for such a structure:

1 Describe the present situation.
2 Explain the factors which may have caused or contributed to the situation at hand.
3 Assess the effects/benefits of the factors/interventions and their consequences.

4 Suggest a programme of improvements leading to confirmation of intended effect or leading to further improvement or development.

These four steps provide a basic framework that can be applied in many forms of evaluations. For example, in the case of a training course on occupational health practice, they can be modified into the following:

1 Describe the effects of the training course.
2 Explain how these effects have been achieved.
3 Assess which effects of the training course are satisfactory, taking into account expectations and earlier agreed requirements.
4 Suggest action to correct deficiencies or to achieve improvements.

This seemingly simple framework has its pitfalls. These are:

• Descriptions may be false, incomplete or even irrelevant.
• Explanations may be more or less plausible.
• Assessments may be inaccurate.
• Suggestions for improvement may be more or less realistic or adequate.

One important element in the planning of an evaluation is to get to know the objectives of the object or activity to be evaluated. On the surface, this may seem a rather self-evident statement. Nevertheless, it is surprisingly often observed that health professionals in a service unit under evaluation do not know or understand the objectives of their own organization. It also happens that even when objectives are known, they are only approximately accepted and pursued. It is also common to encounter health service organizations where there are no explicit objectives for the work being carried out. There are only general, and usually rather vague, indications concerning the general direction of activities.

Having succinct and clearly stated objectives for the activity to be evaluated is of great help to the evaluator. Is there a management objective indicating a desired direction of change? There might, for example, be a shift in emphasis with regard to service output towards preventive services from previously predominantly curative services. In such a case, the evaluation might focus on whether such a change has actually taken place. If, by contrast, the evaluator is expected to describe the full range of services provided by an OHS unit in order to explore customer satisfaction, the evaluation has to be planned in the light of this. The key question, best addressed at an early stage is, 'What is the objective of the evaluation?'

Accordingly, if there are objectives for the performance of services produced by OHS, these should be stated and made subject to examination. What are they? Are they known by the staff?

If the objective of the activity to be evaluated is of a directional character, the evaluation should be designed to provide information or confidence that the processes evaluated actually takes the OHS unit in that direction.

Example: Customer satisfaction with services provided by an OHS unit is to be improved. The first step is to clarify what customer expectations really are, and then to find out whether decisions and steps taken by the unit and other important stakeholders (such as the enterprises involved) really satisfy this requirement. And, if so, how and to what extent?

If the objective is a durable or sustained state of affairs, with specifications of kinds and quantities of service outputs, the evaluation should be planned accordingly.

Example: An OHS unit has the objective of performing one hundred workplace visits in combination with training sessions on emergency first aid. The first elementary step to take by the evaluator is to find out, by examining the records of the service unit, the extent to which this objective has actually been met. If more detailed information is required on the quality of the workplace visit programme, an in-depth survey is necessary.

Example: An OHS unit was assessed with regard to services provided to customer enterprises. In contracts between the unit and the enterprises, objectives were described only in terms of types of service outputs. No specification was made of what the services were supposed to achieve. The external evaluator chose to describe the service items produced in terms of:

- number of consultations;
- types of consultations;
- actions undertaken on the basis of consultations;
- health screening practices – number of pre-employment medical examinations and health surveillance operations;
- number of workplace visits by OHS staff;
- number of training sessions organized by the OHS unit.

Clearly, an evaluation carried out in this manner does not provide information on customers' assessments of the utility value of services, or their satisfaction with the services as such. Nor does it explore interactions between clients and the health organization providing the services to be evaluated.

In performing evaluations of OHS, it is commonly observed that the objectives of the programme evaluated are defined only in terms of types of services provided. The objective is often 'unqualified service delivery', implying that there are no defined end-objectives amenable to evaluation. The utility value of the programmes produced by the OHS unit does not come into question. More often than not, it is not referred to in the written agreement on the evaluation to be carried out.

The object of evaluation

The object of an evaluation or assessment may be poorly specified. It is not clearly stated whether the object is the process as such, i.e. the provision of OHS services, or the effect of the services produced. It sometimes even happens that those who initiate the evaluation have not made up their mind about what the real object is.

Example: The OHS of a large enterprise has, in examining psychological job strain, identified two departments – the marketing and sales department, and the stores department – where complaints are particularly common, and also associated with sickness absenteeism and discontent. An external evaluation team is called in. It is requested by the company to evaluate observations made by OHS.

What is the object of the evaluation in this example?

- The appropriateness of the methods employed by the OHS in the investigation and thereby validity of results?
- Interpretation of the findings of the survey carried out by the OHS unit and the handling of results?
- The action undertaken by the customer and impact of the change?
- The satisfaction of personnel in the two departments with their OHS?
- The utility value of services provided as perceived by the customer?
- The effects on sickness absenteeism, or dissatisfaction of enterprise staff with working conditions?
- An assessment of OHS staff competence and skills in handling the situation, and efficiency in service delivery and utilization of survey results for intervention in the workplace?

As a rule of good practice, it is preferable to have evaluation priorities discussed with the sponsor/customer at the outset. In practice, only a few – sometimes only one or two – objects of evaluation can be explored in depth. The alternative is to accept a wide range of objects, but also to accept that these will necessarily be subject to less comprehensive assessment.

Objectives in evaluation

Objectives in evaluations of OHS are designed to:

- provide a basis for discussion and agreement on the general direction of OHS objectives and service activities;
- facilitate management of OHS work and assessment of resource needs;
- clarify the objects of evaluation in assessing performance and achievements.

The achievement of an organization or an activity is usually one of the most important objects in an evaluation. This issue may be addressed by questions such as:

- In what regards is the organization achieving its objectives?
- What can be done to improve achievement in relation to objectives?
- What can be done to sustain a satisfactory level of achievement?
- How should objectives be conceived in order to make them achievable?

In practice, this means that the first step in an evaluation consists in examining and interpreting the objectives of an organization or service unit. These objectives may be very clear and operational. But they can also be of a more general nature, ambiguous and unrealistic. Also, they may originally have been written for the purposes of information, or for marketing of services, not to provide a basis for evaluation. Key questions are:

- What objectives have been set?
- How tangible or visible is the achievement of objectives, i.e. how do professional staff or customers become aware that the organization is achieving what it has set out to achieve?

These are questions that generate discussions with management and staff of evaluated units, which may then provide information on issues to bring into focus, including ambiguities and disagreements. General experience is that it is much easier to know and to describe ongoing OHS activities than the actual objectives these activities are designed to achieve.

Different types of objectives

There are different types of objectives of OHS organizations, which should be kept separate in planning an evaluation. These are:

- service objectives – output of services (workplace health promotion, rehabilitation of injured staff, health service programmes, risk assessments etc.);
- activity objectives – effects or impact of services (improvement of health of individuals or groups of staff in client enterprises, reduction in sickness absenteeism, incidence of work injuries etc.);
- training objectives – development of skills (knowledge, competencies etc.) among staff of client enterprises or own OHS unit;
- structural objectives – efficient organization (e.g. reappraisal and redistribution of responsibilities and work tasks);
- method objectives – improvement in efficiency and quality of processes (workplace or work-organization investigation techniques, pedagogics in training programmes, structuring of contacts in specified preventive operations etc.);
- personnel objectives – work satisfaction, social support and relations (interaction between members of OHS professional staff, feedback in management etc.).

Data collection and measurement

In planning for the collection of information and data, it is important to remember that there is an intimate relationship between objectives and objects of an evaluation on the one hand and methods to be used on the other. No method or measurement is, as a matter of principle, superior to others. It all depends on what the evaluator is setting out to achieve.

Evaluations of health services in general and of OHS in particular may – as has been described above – apply different concepts, and focus on various and differing aspects of the service unit or activity to be evaluated. This has implications for the selection of methods, measures of performance, and comparisons. Assessments and measurements of performance are usually made in terms of:

- activity (e.g. number of individual consultations, investigations of work conditions, workplace visits, number of staff participating in health-surveillance schemes etc.);
- costs/resource consumption (e.g. unit costs, consultations costs, costs of health examinations, administrative costs, computer costs);
- inputs/structure (e.g. number and type of staff, organizational roles and management structure);
- process (e.g. delays and waiting times, quality indicators, perceived efficiency);
- outputs (e.g. number of individual rehabilitation programmes, staff covered by occupational health training sessions, risk assessment consultations);
- outcome (morbidity and impact on perceived health and well-being, client satisfaction, impact on resource use, initiation of preventive action, such as workplace interventions).

The issues to be considered in making performance assessments include clearly defining the entity of measurement and unit of performance (e.g. exactly which service item or product is being assessed). Does the same entity of measurement apply throughout the range of contexts in which services are provided by the OHS unit?

The next question is which aspect of performance will be considered:

- economy – fewest resources or lowest cost (input);
- productivity – amount produced (output);
- efficiency – input/output relationship;
- effectiveness – how well the service achieves desired results, i.e. change effected in the target, or how well it meets objectives defined at outset;
- quality – the degree to which the services satisfy clients' needs and meet professionally defined requirements.

It is important to select measures and to make observations for assessment of performances or outcomes that meet the following requirements:

- The measures and observations performed should be pertinent to the key questions selected as points of departure for designing the evaluation.
- The measures and observations should help the people who gather the data to improve their performance.
- The measures and observations should help assess something that can be changed.

Types of evaluation

A distinction is usually made between formative and summative evaluations. The purpose of a **formative evaluation** is to give to the organizations and persons involved in an evaluation (i.e. both evaluators and those evaluated) information and support with a view to developing and improving their performance. This may cover clarification of aims, awareness and understanding of the attitudes and demands of customers/clients, and differences between stated intentions and everyday practice.

A **summative evaluation** aims primarily at helping managers and other decision-makers to assess the effects and efficiency of programmes/projects with a view to deciding whether it should be continued or abandoned, or modified. The focus of summative evaluations is most often on outcomes and outputs of service products. They are usually designed to satisfy external stakeholders' interests.

Process evaluation is most often performed with a formative purpose, but it may also be carried out with a summative intention. It is carried out when the outcomes and effects of a programme or action taken lie in the future – sometimes with considerable delay – with the implication that an evaluation is advisable before they eventually materialize. A process evaluation focuses on programmes and activities that are already well under way. Processes, procedures and tasks are examined at an OHS unit in the course of its work. A process evaluation addresses questions such as:

- What are the stated aims and objectives of the different service components?
- Who is served by what type of service?
- How is the service delivered and what does it consist of?
- What are the quality indicators?
- What happens in the course of service provision?
- What is the interaction between the service provider and the customer?

The other principal and often performed type of evaluation is the **outcome evaluation.** It may target short-term outcomes that are immediately observable, such as changes in persons, customer groups and workplaces. This may concern knowledge, awareness, behaviour, risk assessment, or management. It may also target more long-term types of effects, such as changes in work organization, procedures and work practices, or health outcomes in the enterprise or corporation. Outcome evaluations are often planned as summative evaluations, since they focus on the effects and outputs of a service unit. The effects or outcomes studied in outcome evaluations may be of either the expected or intended type (or both), and they may also be undertaken with regard to unexpected effects of a programme. Summative evaluations of outcome may include:

- changes in attitudes and knowledge and behaviour, including health behaviour;
- changes in health status or self-rated health as assessed on the basis of criteria defined by health professionals;
- changes in morbidity or mortality;
- changes in company occupational health policies and practices;

- effects on work organization or stakeholders, or relations to stake-holders in a broad sense.

In practice, evaluations are often carried out with a blend of summative and formative intentions. For example, a summative assessment may move into a formative phase – with the aim of improving efficiency, productivity or quality standards.

The terms 'outcome' and 'impact' are sometimes used interchangeably in descriptions of evaluation procedures, since it is conceptually difficult to keep them apart. In this book, **outcome** denotes evaluation of what has occurred as a result of an OHS programme or action. It refers to success or non-success in both programmes of short or long duration, and it includes assessments of results or achievements in relation to previously defined aims or expectations. **Impact** denotes, in the same way, evaluation of the effects a programme has had on an organization and on important stakeholders. But an impact evaluation goes a bit further than an outcome evaluation in that it also assesses or measures the changes in an organization, or its functionings or practices, resulting from outcomes effected.

Preparing for and proceeding with an evaluation

In preparing for an evaluation, the following steps need to be taken:

- Define aims and objectives of the evaluation.
- Settle the arena of the evaluation (internal to the OHS unit evaluated, internal to an enterprise or company, arena extending outside unit or company, public arena).
- Familiarize yourself with the documentary system and records of the OHS organization to be evaluated.
- Specify outcomes and indicators of success or, as appropriate, non-success.
- Define the activities or programme components to be evaluated.
- In analytic studies, assess the credibility of the linkage between evaluated activities and stated outcomes.
- Develop a work plan, budget and time plan for the evaluation.
- Nominate or select an evaluation team.
- Plan for, and structure, contacts with evaluated service representatives, with stakeholders, and within the evaluation team.

Consider the following steps in making a work plan (which includes a budget/resource plan and time plan):

- Design evaluation procedure.
- Examine documents on objectives, organization, functions, procedures, methods and routines of the OHS unit, including training and skills development of OHS staff.
- Develop data collection tools and explore information sources to be used.
- Organize pilot data collection runs utilizing the methods to be employed.

- Collect data and make observations.
- Analyse observations made and data collected.
- Draft report.
- Communicate and disseminate results and report.

Know what you are trying to achieve

In defining aims and objectives, it is important to define what the programme to be evaluated is designed to achieve.

It is equally important to identify the specific and measurable outcomes that are related to the programme objective. Is the objective of the programme an implementation, i.e. something which is done, or is it an outcome objective, i.e. an effect?

An implementation objective might be:

- provision of a health-screening programme for a department in a customer enterprise where there are particular workplace health hazards;
- providing, say, fifteen one-day training sessions for emergency first aid in a group of customer enterprises.

Outcome objectives refer to the results that are to be expected or to be achieved in the course of an occupational health activity. Examples are:

- obtaining 80% satisfaction ratings among persons undergoing programmes for rehabilitation-counselling services;
- a 50% decrease in serious accidents in a particularly risk-prone department of an enterprise or category of staff.

In measuring rates of satisfaction, it should be observed that a target group in the staff population has to be defined, and then approached with questions through questionnaires or interviews. In measuring the impact of accident-prevention programmes, it is necessary to know the situation before the preventive action was taken.

Success indicators are important tools. For each outcome objective there should be well-defined and practically usable success indicator(s) to help determine whether a programme is successful or not. Success indicators show:

- whether you achieve what you set out to do;
- what may be considered as effective;
- what is meant by a success.

If objectives have been well defined, this is helpful in identifying success indicators. It is significantly more difficult if objectives have not been defined.

Examples of measurable indicators

Formative evaluations:

- service utilization;
- delays in service delivery;

- occupational health professionals' perceptions of needs of populations served;
- customers' and stakeholders' perception of needs in populations served;
- risk assessments.

Process evaluations:

- OHS staff-time input;
- expenditures;
- costs;
- customer participation;
- complaints and enquiries;
- priority setting;
- training sessions;
- information activities;
- risk assessments.

Outcome evaluations:

- policy changes in occupational health programmes;
- changes in customer awareness and expertise in occupational health matters;
- benefits to customers, staff or management;
- change in volume of service provided, or type and quality of service;
- changes in utilization of occupational health services;
- changes in behaviour of customer groups, professional staff and management;
- morbidity/mortality;
- health or health indicators.

In preparing an evaluation of a programme, an important step is to become familiar with the target population of the occupational health programme being evaluated. This implies collection of information on basic demographic facts, such as age and gender. In addition, socio-economic information, e.g. on educational qualifications, is needed – as too is detailed information on occupations, work organization, work tasks and work conditions. Other relevant information may be the geographic distribution of the target population, which affects how best to communicate with its members.

Involving stakeholders

An evaluation practically always involves many 'stakeholders'. The term refers to all those persons or organizations that need to be involved in, or may be affected by, an OHS evaluation. Accordingly, one essential step in such an evaluation is to identify the stakeholders who might be interested in the evaluation findings, and what their interests and expectations are. The measures to take are as follows:

- Identify stakeholders of the programme to be evaluated.
- Identify stakeholders of the evaluation.

- Assess stakeholders' expectations and information needs.
- Plan for contacts with stakeholder groups.

It is also important to establish the roles of the various stakeholders. Some evaluations may entail a need to involve stakeholders from the planning and decision-making stages of the evaluation process, while the role of others may imply active participation in the actual conduct of the evaluation. An evaluator is usually well advised to assume that most stakeholders will wish to participate and be involved in all aspects of an evaluation project. In considerations of stakeholder roles and involvement, it is important to pay attention to aspects of confidentiality. Some information and observations made during the evaluation may need to be regarded as company-confidential.

In evaluations of OHS, the obvious important stakeholders are the employers and the employees, and their respective organizations. OHS professionals make up another important stakeholder category. Public stakeholders may be government agencies, community services and insurance companies, or social-security agencies. Well-carried-out stakeholder identification – with structuring of contacts before, during and after evaluation – is often one of the key prerequisites for a successful evaluation project.

Evaluation design

Designing an evaluation means selecting the type of evaluation to be conducted. When deciding on design, the following questions need to be considered:

- What are the key questions to be answered in the course of the evaluation?
- How long has the programme to be evaluated been in operation?
- What is the state of development of the programme to be evaluated?
- Have there been previous evaluations?
- What stakeholders are involved, and what are their interests?

Once objectives and type of evaluation have been decided upon, the next step is to consider evaluation design. Basically, depending on the key questions to be addressed and evaluation needs, a descriptive design approach or, alternatively, an analytic approach, seeking explanations to what has been observed, may be required. Most formative and process evaluations are descriptive by nature, and do not require an experimental design or measurements before and after intervention.

Analytic outcome evaluations require a design demonstrating that the action or programme under study has had the intended outcome. This is a more sophisticated design requirement, and the reader is referred to John Øvretveit's chapter on intervention evaluation in this book (Chapter 4).

As a general principle, descriptive studies are concerned with describing the general characteristics of the population under study, the workplaces involved, and the relevant features of the work environment, the organization of work and the programmes of the OHS being evaluated.

Descriptive evaluations are the most commonly used. They are usually less demanding than evaluations designed to analyse relationships between causal factors and effects. Also, they are usually less expensive. An evaluator is well advised to start with an overview description. It may be conducted as a case study, which is the most basic type of evaluation design. The study describes the target population and the programme, its characteristics and its effects or outcomes. In terms of the time dimension, the description may be at one point of time, or of a process over a lengthy period.

Analytic studies go beyond the simple description of characteristics. Their objective is usually to explain the phenomena and events that have been described in a preceding descriptive study, which has suggested causal relationships between OHS actions and important outcomes. They may involve a comparison between groups in order to determine, for example, whether or not an intervention has had an effect, or whether one intervention programme is more effective than another. In analytically designed programmes, the evaluator usually resorts to a control technique enabling comparisons to be made between target groups subject to different interventions, e.g. between index groups and groups subject to no intervention at all. In real life, evaluations designed as a true experiment are very rare – due to both ethical and technical constraints. In practice, evaluations carried out with an analytic objective often have to limit themselves to a quasi-experimental design.

Qualitative and quantitative methods

In deciding how to collect the information needed to evaluate an occupational health programme or activity, selection of method or methods is important. Basically, the evaluator has to choose between qualitative and quantitative methods, or a blend of these two approaches. Which should be chosen is determined by the objective of the evaluation, the key questions providing the basis for the evaluation, and the design selected as suitable for the task.

Qualitative methods

The qualitative methodological approach implies direct observations, exploratory interviews, in-depth interviews, open-ended questions in surveys, or use of diaries and discussions in focus groups. The information derived and analysed leads to a comprehensive and, depending on time and effort, detailed description of the object or activity under study. The spotlight is on what is characteristic of the examined organization, including its environment and context, without there necessarily being a preconceived idea of how the phenomena observed are to be explained. No hypotheses are usually required at the first exploratory stages of a qualitative evaluation. It is assumed that the important and unique features of the organization under study will surface through combining observations of many different kinds.

Quantitative methods

The quantitative method aims at defining in numeric terms a qualitative characteristic of an organization or a process. This may, for example, concern rates or numbers of accidents, levels of noise in the workplace, customer satisfaction as expressed in mailed questionnaire responses, results obtained in structured interviews, number of workplace visits carried out by OHS professionals, or direct measurements of physical or biochemical characteristics of workplaces or populations served by an OHS organization. Analysis of registered information on sickness absence at aggregate level in personnel records is another type of quantitative method. The spotlight is on what is typical, representative or common with regard to the quality being assessed. The use of quantitative methods assumes that the phenomena under study possess in principle the same qualities – accepting that the measured or assessed value may, for some items, be recorded as zero. Before opting for quantitative methods of assessment, it is necessary to decide which qualitative aspects of the organization or activity studied are important to assess (in view of the objectives of the evaluation), and to review the methods available for use. This also includes taking into account issues of design, such as sampling and representativeness. Issues of validity, including sensitivity, specificity and relevance of methods, also have to be examined in selecting suitable quantitative methods.

The relationship between the evaluator and the object, whether an organization or an activity being assessed, often differs according to whether qualitative or quantitative methods are adopted. Use of the qualitative method usually implies a close contact between the evaluator and those being assessed – ranging from the evaluator acting as an observer through to even actively participating in the process examined. Procedures are commonly of a non-standard nature, and the number of subjects under observation is limited. By contrast, the evaluator using primarily quantitative methods assumes a more distant relationship to those evaluated, in that data derived in a standard way from – usually – a large number of subjects are analysed.

The subject of qualitative versus quantitative methods will not be elaborated further in this book. In general, however, it can be said that qualitative methods generate detailed in-depth information on just a few subjects. The results are not, and do not claim to be, generalizable to entire populations. Quantitative methods generate structured data from greater numbers of subjects, and are designed to achieve generalizable results with validity external to the subjects examined. This means that in selecting between qualitative and quantitative methods in evaluation it is essential to look at the problem or question to be addressed. If a comprehensive understanding of the functioning of an organization is sought, including social processes, qualitative methods are usually good starters. If however, when studying a sample of observations or phenomena, information is sought on what is representative in the sampling frame or feature under study, quantitative methods may be better suited. This also applies if the objective is to make comparisons between observed organizations in some specific regard. For more detailed discussions of these methodological issues, the reader is referred to the standard textbooks included among some of the bibliographic references following each chapter in this book. The strengths and weaknesses of these two categories of methods have been summarized by The Health Communication Unit Centre for Health Promotion of the University of Toronto, Ontario, Canada (1998) as follows:

Strengths and weaknesses of different methods of measurement

(These are some of the qualitative and quantitative methods)

Qualitative methods	*Quantitative methods*
A Focus groups	G Intercept, mail or telephone survey
B In-depth interviews	H Process tracking forms/records
C Open-ended survey questions	I Service utilization
D Diaries	J Analysis of large datasets
E Consensus building (Delphi method)	K Direct measures of health (Delphi method) (indicators/ behaviours, e.g. blood pressure)
F Forums/discussion groups	L Direct measures of illness (mortality/morbidity rates)

To determine what methods should be used, match them to:

- the programme's success indicators;
- the resources available;
- the best way to collect information from the population of interest.

You need to determine:

- the best way to communicate with participants (telephone, mail?);
- when to communicate with them (daytime, evenings?);
- how to limit burden on them.

In concluding this chapter, we wish to emphasize that the methods selected in the course of an evaluation process have no life of their own. They are determined by the definition of the evaluation problem, the objective of the planned assessment, the frame of questions to be addressed in the course of an evaluation, and the evaluation design. For some purposes, structured interviews may be adequate, whereas, for others, quantitative information on occupational health or field-survey projects may be more relevant. Often, a combination of qualitative and quantitative methods is selected, such as open interviews supplemented by structured questionnaires.

Bibliography

Davies, J.K. and Macdonald, G. (eds) (1998) *Quality, Evidence and Effectiveness in Health Promotion – Striving for Certainties.* London: Routledge.
Denzin, N.K. and Lincoln, Y.S. (eds) (1994) *Handbook of Qualitative Research.* Thousand Oaks, CA: Sage Publications.

Haglund, B., Jansson, B., Pettersson, B. *et al*. (1998) Methods for assessing quality. In: *Quality, Evidence and Effectiveness in Health Promotion – Striving for Certainties* (Davies, J.K. and MacDonald, G., eds) London: Routledge.

Health Communication Unit Centre for Health Promotion (1998), *Evaluating Health Promotion Programmes*. The Banting Institute, University of Toronto Publications.

Joint Committee on Standards for Educational Evaluation (ed. J.R. Sanders, Chair) (1994) *The Program Evaluation Standards*, 2nd edn, Thousand Oaks, CA: Sage Publications.

Øvretveit, J. (1998) *Evaluating Health Interventions*. Buckingham: Open University Press.

8

International comparison highlights the standards of OHS – the Japanese case

Takashi Muto

Japanese occupational health services (OHS) were examined from an international comparative perspective in order to highlight current problems and suggest possible improvements. Three sets of documents were used to illustrate the characteristics of Japanese OHS. The OHS Recommendation of the ILO was employed as an international comparative standard. The analysis was organized according to the conceptual framework developed by Donabedian (1988) that distinguishes between structure, process and outcome. Specific potential difficulties were found with regard to type of organization (in particular with regard to small-scale enterprises), function of nurses, quantity and quality of training, coverage for the self-employed and ambiguity of clinical role. Very little information on the outcomes of OHS activities was available. As a formal-documentation-based study, issues of implementation were not addressed.

Development of OHS in Japan

In recent years, there have been a number of substantial changes in occupational health practice in Japan (although surprisingly little discussion of paths to take for the future). The Japan Medical Association started an accreditation system for qualified occupational physicians in 1990 (JMA, 1990). The Japan Society for Occupational Health initiated board certification for certified occupational physicians in 1992 (JSOH, 1994), and qualifications were awarded to physicians who passed the relevant examination. In 1993, the Ministry of Labour adopted a new policy aimed at improving occupational health services (OHS) in small-scale enterprises (SSEs) (MOL, 1994). There is a plan to establish occupational health centres (OHCs) at regional and prefectural levels throughout the country within the next seven years. From 1992 to 1994, several proposals were made with regard to an ideal OHS system for Japan (SCIFOP, 1992; JFEA, 1993; MOL, 1995a). Following these proposals, the Safety and Health Act was revised in May 1996, with amendments coming into force in October 1996 (MOL, 1996). The changes suggest that improvements in OHS in Japan were needed in several respects.

OHS in Japan have been scrutinized by a number of researchers

(Tsuchiya, 1991; Higashi *et al.*, 1994; Takahashi and Okubo, 1994; Muto *et al.*, 1995a; Mizoue *et al.*, 1996; Okubo, 1997, 1998), but few studies have compared Japanese OHS with those of other countries. One study evaluated the current problems of Japanese OHS by means of comparison with the ILO Convention and Recommendation (Okubo, 1994). However, it assessed only current measures taken by OHS in Japan, and did not take into account discussions concerning any future, and possibly more desirable, Japanese OHS systems. Accordingly, the current status and future scope of Japanese OHS have not so far been systematically examined from an international perspective. This study was conducted to clarify the problems of current Japanese OHS from precisely this viewpoint.

Documentary base for the comparative evaluation

Three documents (or sets of documents) were used to illustrate the characteristics of Japanese OHS:

- The first was the Industrial Safety and Health Act (ISH Act), revised in 1996, and relevant accompanying legislation – in particular the Cabinet Order and Ministry of Labour Ordinance (MOL, 1995b; MOL, 1996). This legislation is described as the 'ISH Law' for the purposes of this study. It should be noted that the ISH Law forms the legislative core of current occupational health practice in Japan, and was selected for analysis precisely on this ground.
- The second was the Report of the Study Committee on the Ideal Functions of Occupational Physicians (SCIFOP, 1992). The committee was organized by the director of the Labour Standard Bureau of the Ministry of Labour, and submitted its report in 1992. The report was selected for analysis largely because OHS are discussed broadly therein (despite the fact that the more limited primary remit of the committee was to investigate the ideal functions of occupational physicians). The report consists of two parts – thirteen proposals, plus accounts of the discussions underlying these proposals. Note that opinions in the discussion part are also examined in this study.
- The third was the Report of the Study Committee on the Ideal Method of Promoting Occupational Health (MOL, 1995a). This committee was also organized by the director of the Labour Standard Bureau of the Ministry of Labour, and submitted its report in 1994. The report was selected mainly because OHS needs for the twenty-first century were discussed.

Since the two committees (for Ideal Functions of Occupational Physicians, and for Ideal Method of Promoting Occupational Health) were considered to be complementary, their opinions are set forth as those of 'the Committee' in the comparisons that follow.

Two possible international standards for comparison were considered:

- the 1985 Occupational Health Services Recommendation of the ILO and accompanying Recommendation No. 171 (ILO, 1985);
- WHO's 1990 *Occupational Health Services: an Overview* (Rantanen, 1990).

Although the ILO recommendation predated the WHO overview, the former was selected on the grounds that it contained the most authoritative list of the functions of OHS, and also provided a good point of reference for inter-country comparisons.

The analysis was conducted using a conceptual framework developed by Donabedian (1988), which encompasses the terms, structure, process and outcome. Structure refers to the resources available for providing health care – organization, facilities and the types and qualifications of professionals in the field. Process refers to the performance of these professionals in terms of meeting accepted standards – access to care, rate of utilization, protocol for the evaluation of OHS, and so on. Outcomes are defined as the end results of health care – including health status, improvement of function, longevity, comfort and quality of life.

With regard to the particular case of SSEs, four principles of occupational health administration used by the Japanese Ministry of Labour in Japan were adopted as a framework of evaluation (see Muto, 1995a):

- surveillance and control of the work environment;
- improvement of working methods;
- health evaluation;
- health education.

These four principles were regarded as OHS process functions within the Donabedian framework, one that is broader than that of the Ministry of Labour. Current and future Japanese OHS were categorized according to the following standards (the upper-case letters referring to entries in the 'Judgement' column in Tables 8.1–8.3.

- Not stated or specified in the ILO, but stated or specified in the ISH Law or Committee reports (A).
- Stated or specified both in the ILO and in the ISH Law or Committee reports (B).
- Stated in the ILO, but not stated or specified in the ISH Law or Committee reports (C).

The results of the international comparisons are presented in the form of tables and accompanying observations organized under subheadings of the three main categories – structure, process and outcome.

Observations on OHS structure

Organization

The ILO proposed five possible organizations of OHS – (joint) undertakings, public authorities, social-security institutions, and so on. But no concrete organizational forms are mentioned either in the ISH Law or by the Committee. The revised ISH Law stipulates that a safety and health committee is established at each workplace in companies employing 50 or more workers. By contrast, the Committee proposed that such a committee is established at each workplace in which 30 or more workers are employed.

With regard to SSEs, it was envisaged that OHS might be organized as a service common to a number of undertakings (according to the ILO Recommendation). The ISH Law states that special consideration should be given to SSEs in conducting financial and technical assistance with respect to the implementation of safety and health measures taken by employers. The Committee recommended the establishment of regional occupational health centres for SSEs. Further, in order to secure workers' privacy and enable objective judgements independent of employer or employees, certain standards of 'fairness' should apply within any enterprise.

Premises and facilities

The ILO specifies that OHS units should be located within or near the place of employment, or should be organized in such a way as to ensure that OHS functions are carried out at the place of employment. The Committee stated that premises for OHS may be in-house or external.

The ILO specifies that OHS should have access to appropriate facilities for carrying out the analyses and tests necessary for surveillance of workers' health and the work environment. The Committee mentioned that facilities for OHS should be provided for the 'convenience' of workers.

Staffing

The ILO specifies that OHS should have sufficient technical personnel with specialized training and experience in fields such as occupational medicine, occupational health nursing, occupational hygiene and ergonomics. While figures regarding the number of occupational physicians required are not given by the ILO, both the ISH Law and the Committee lay down a concrete figure. The ISH Law stipulates that a physician

Table 8.1 *Comparison of OHS structures in terms of organization and facilities*

Focus	ILO Recommendation No.171	ISH Law	Committee Report	Judgement
		Japan		
Organization				
Organization model	5 organizations	NS	NS	C
S&H committee	Stated but not specified	No.emp >50	No. emp >30	B
Measures for SSEs	Organized	Special consideration	Occupational health centre	B
Fairness	NS	NS	Should be kept	A
Facilities				
Premises	Within/near workplace	NS	In-house or external	B
Facilities	Should be accessed	NS	For the convenience of workers	B

NS, Not stated.
A, Not stated or specified in the ILO, but stated or specified in the ISH Law or Committee reports.
B, Stated or specified both in the ILO and in the ISH Law or Committee reports.
C, Stated or specified in the ILO, but not stated or specified in the ISH Law or Committee reports.

should be assigned to any workplace where more than 50 workers are employed. The Committee proposed that the number of employees should be 30 instead of 50. Further, it was proposed that a specified time (hours per week) of access to an occupational health physician at workplaces should be prescribed with the aim to secure satisfactory occupational health care.

There were no legal provisions concerning qualification of occupational physicians in the earlier ISH Law, but the revised Law stipulates that they must have 'sufficient knowledge' to provide occupational health care for workers. The proposal with regard to qualification in the Committee reports is very similar.

Formerly, there were no legal requirements for working as a nurse in OHS. It was enough to be a nurse of some kind. In the revised ISH Law, the functions of 'health nurses' were stipulated for the first time. The nurses are to provide health guidance for employees requiring assistance in maintaining their health. The Committee recommended that use is made of both health nurses and nurses.

In the ISH Law, there are no stipulations concerning ergonomists, industrial hygienists, or administrative personnel. But there are now legal definitions of the functions of industrial health consultants and work environment measurement experts (in the ISH Law and Work Environment Measurement Law, respectively). Industrial health consultants (mostly experienced occupational physicians), health supervisors or health nurses holding a licence issued by the Ministry of Labour are entitled to provide health consultancy in the workplace at the request of the employer.

Work environment measurements must be carried out by experts holding a specialized licence from the Ministry of Labour. The Committee recommended that such personnel be employed in OHS. More specifically, the ISH Law stipulates that workers who handle acids should be examined by a dentist. The Committee proposed the promotion of oral health through the assistance of dentists and dental hygienists in the workplace.

According to the ISH Law, all workplaces with 100 or more workers are obliged to appoint a general safety and health director, and all those with 50 or more, a health supervisor. The general safety and health director – usually a factory or branch manager – would exercise general control over the workplace. Health supervisors, who are licensed by the chief of the Prefectural Labour Standards Office, take charge of technical matters related to health in the workplace. The number of health supervisors needed in each workplace is determined by its size. All workplaces with 10–49 workers are obliged to appoint a health promoter whose responsibilities are almost the same as those of health supervisors. Heath supervisors and health promoters are expected to play an active role as coordinators in OHS.

Further, it is stipulated in the ISH Law and recommended by the Committee that personnel involved in the occupational health arena include health educators, mental health advisers, dieticians and health care trainers. These are new professions, created for the implementation of health promotion programmes in the workplace.

Table 8.2 Comparison of OHS structures in terms of staffing

Focus	ILO Recommendation No.171	Japan		
		ISH Law	Committee Report	Judgement
Occupational physicians	Trained/expertise	Trained physician	Trained physician	B
	Should be staffed	No. emp >50	No. emp >30	
		No. emp >1000 (full)	No. emp >1000 (full)	
		Appointed in the workplace	Based on consumed time	
Occupational-health nurses	Should be staffed	Engage in health guidance	Should be involved	B
Ergonomists	Should be staffed	NS	Should be staffed	B
Industrial hygienists	Should be staffed	NS	Should be staffed	B
Industrial health consultants	NS	Occupational health consultation	Should be utilized	A
Work environment measurement experts	NS	Functions implied	Should be staffed	A
Administrative personnel	Should be staffed	NS	Should be staffed	B
Dentists	NS	In case of harmful work	Should be involved	A
Dental hygienists	NS	NS	Should be involved	A
General safety & health directors	NS	No. emp >100–1000	NS	A
Health supervisors	NS	No. emp >50	Should be active	A
Health promoters	NS	No. emp. 10–49	Should be active	A
Health educators	NS	Should be staffed	Should be staffed	A
Mental health advisers	NS	Should be staffed	Should be staffed	A
Dietitians	NS	Should be staffed	Should be staffed	A
Trainers	NS	Should be staffed	Should be staffed	A
Professional independence	Should be safeguarded	NS	Should be safeguarded	B
Training	Should be given	NS	Should be given	B
Remuneration	NS	NS	Reasonable	A

NS, Not stated.
A, Not stated or specified in the ILO, but stated or specified in the ISH Law or Committee reports.
B, Stated or specified both in the ILO and in the ISH Law or Committee reports.
C, Stated or specified in the ILO, but not stated or specified in the ISH Law or Committee reports.

According to the ILO, the professional independence of OHS personnel should be safeguarded. Nothing was included in the ISH Law regarding such independence, but there is a mention of it in the Committee reports. The Committee advised that occupational staff be given an opportunity to receive education and training. Regarding remuneration, the Committee stated that reasonable remuneration should be provided for occupational physicians. However, neither the ILO nor the ISH Law refers to the issue of remuneration for OHS personnel.

Observations on OHS process

Target groups

Regarding coverage of the working population by OHS, both the ILO and the Committee recommend that all workers are covered. By contrast, the ISH Law refers more narrowly to workers employed at enterprises or places of businesses.

The Committee recommended specific measures for female workers, disabled workers, aged workers, expatriates and foreign workers. The ILO recommends that workers' families are covered by OHS, but they are not covered in Japan.

Functions

The ILO stipulates that the role of OHS should be essentially preventive. The ISH Law stipulates six responsibilities of an occupational physician, all of which are preventive by nature:

• management of work environments;
• management of working methods;
• health care management;
• health examinations;
• health education, hygiene education;
• examination of work-related diseases.

Both the ILO document and the ISH Law contain provisions concerning the surveillance of the work environment and control of methods of work. Promotion of comfortable workplaces is referred to in the ISH Law and by the Committee. It is stipulated by all three parties that appropriate job assignment should be considered or promoted. Health promotion is specified as necessary in the ISH Law and also in the Committee reports.

All three parties also make statements concerning the surveillance of workers' health. But cancer screening is referred to only in the Committee reports, and immunization only by the ILO. The ILO specifies that treatment, including rehabilitation, should be provided. In the ISH Law, however, there are no provisions regarding either treatment or rehabilitation. Nor was any mention of treatment or rehabilitation made by the Committee, although it did refer to measures involving mental health, work-related diseases and AIDS/HIV.

Management

All three parties specify that an activity plan or programme should be established and adopted by OHS. Regarding privacy, the ILO specifies that 'personal data relating to health assessments may be communicated to others only with the informed consent of the worker concerned', and that 'each person who works in an OHS should be required to observe professional secrecy as regards both medical and technical information'. All three parties share the opinion that each worker should be informed of the results of personal health examinations and assessments of his/her health.

Regarding reporting to the employer, the ILO specifies that 'the physician who has carried out the examination should communicate his conclusions in writing to both the worker and the employer'. The ISH Law stipulates that recommendations by an occupational physician to the employer should be respected. ILO stated that an occupational disease detected through workers' health surveillance should be notified to the competent authority in accordance with national law and practice. The ISH Law stated that the results of health examinations are to be reported to the chief of a Labour Standards Inspection Office.

Concerning record keeping, the ILO specifies that 'OHS should record data on workers' health in personal confidential health files'. The ILO also states that 'the conditions under which, and time during which, personal health files should be kept, should be prescribed by national laws'. The ISH Law stipulates that the employer must keep records of the results of medical examinations for a period of five years.

According to the ILO, OHS units should be encouraged to contribute to research by participating in studies (in their undertakings) with a view to collecting data for epidemiological purposes and orienting their activities. The Committee states that basic research on health should be promoted. Cooperation with community health services is specifically referred to both in the ILO document and by the Committee.

Observations on OHS outcomes

Very little was mentioned by any of the three parties concerning outcomes of OHS activities. The Committee specified that economic evaluations should be conducted, implying financial outcome should be one of the evaluation standards employed.

Concluding remarks

Several characteristics of Japanese OHS have been clarified by the study.

First, with regard to structure of OHS, there is no uniform type of OHS organization in Japan. Currently, there are at least three types of OHS in large enterprises – company-owned OHS, OHS managed by health insurance societies, and OHS managed by a subsidiary organization within a company (Muto et al., 1995b). In the case of SSEs, there are

Table 8.3 *Comparison of OHS process*

| Focus | ILO Recommendation No.171 | Japan | | Judgement |
		ISH Law	Committee Report	
Target				
Coverage	All workers	Employed workers	All workers	B
Self-employed	Should be available	NS	NS	C
Female workers	NS	NS	Should be promoted	A
Disabled workers	NS	NS	Should be promoted	A
Aged workers	NS	Should be promoted	Should be promoted	A
Expatriates	NS	Health examination	Should be promoted	A
Foreign workers	NS	NS	Should be promoted	A
Workers families	Should be provided	NS	NS	C
Functions				
Role of OHS	Preventive	Ensuring safety & health	Promotion of health	B
Environmental surveillance	Specified	Specified	Should be conducted	B
Methods of work	Specified	Specified	Specified	B
Comfortable workplace	NS	Should be promoted	Should be promoted	A
Job assignment	Should be considered	Should be promoted	Should be promoted	B
Health promotion	NS	Should be promoted	Should be promoted	A
Health surveillance	Specified	Specified	Specified	B
Cancer screening	NS	NS	Should be promoted	A
Immunization	Might be carried out	NS	NS	C
Treatment	Possible	NS	NS	C
Rehabilitation	Should be undertaken	NS	NS	C
Mental health	NS	Should be promoted	Should be promoted	A
Work-related disease	NS	NS	Should be promoted	A
AIDS/HIV	NS	NS	Should be promoted	A

Table 8.3 (*Continued*)

			Japan	
Focus	*ILO Recommendation No.171*	*ISH Law*	*Committee Report*	*Judgement*
Management				
Programme of activity	Should be established	Should be adopted	Should be involved	B
Personal health data	Should be protected	Should be protected	Should be protected	B
Report to employee	Be informed	Should be informed	Should be informed	B
Recommendation to employer	Should be done	Should be respected	Should be respected	B
Report to competent authority	Should be done	Must be done	NS	B
Record keeping	Should record	5 years	Certain period	B
Research	Contribute	NS	Be promoted	B
Continuous care	NS	NS	ID card	A
Community health	Collaboration	NS	Collaboration	B

NS, Not stated.
A, Not stated or specified in the ILO, but stated or specified in the ISH Law or Committee reports.
B, Stated or specified both in the ILO and in the ISH Law or Cond in the ISH Law or Committee reports.
C, Stated or specified in the ILO, but not stated or specified in the ISH Law or Committee reports.

multiple OHS channels, each with characteristics of their own (Muto *et al.*, 1995a). The pros and cons of these organizations should be investigated, in the first instance in order to identify the most efficient type of organization. Under current circumstances, it can be imagined that standards for premises and facilities are qualitative rather than quantitative by nature.

Second, except with regard to occupational physicians and health supervisors, staffing standards are generally qualitative. Functions of occupational health nurses are very limited (Muto *et al.*, 1998). The reports recommended that health personnel in charge of health-promotion programmes (such as health educators, mental health advisers, dieticians and trainers) should obtain staff positions, but lack of such personnel ranked as the top reason for not implementing this kind of programme (Muto *et al.*, 1995c). In addition, the quality of health personnel poses a problem. For example, provided that a person has majored in psychology, social welfare or health science in college, he or she can be certified as a mental health adviser even after a 3-day training course. Certification as a counsellor, on the other hand, requires more than one year.

Third, regarding the process of OHS, Japanese OHS does not cover self-employed workers, including farmers and fishermen. The Ministry of Agriculture, Forestry and Fisheries is in charge of prevention of occupational injuries and diseases in these industries. Considering that approximately 400 farmers, mostly elderly ones, are killed by accidents during their work each year (MAFF, 1996), appropriate measures need to be taken in OHS.

Fourth, nothing is mentioned in the reports concerning clinical services. In France and Germany, occupational physicians cannot provide curative treatment (Kroon *et al.*, 1991), but in Japan, there are many companies that provide curative services within the confines of OHS. One company, however, has ceased to provide curative services at its health care centre in order to increase the efficiency of OHS (Osaka Gas, 1996). Whether clinical services should be provided by OHS should be openly discussed.

By contrast with those for structure and process, there seem to be very few standards for outcomes. Outcome standards need to be established for quality assurance to be possible. Finally, it should be noted that this study examined only the framework of OHS in terms of structure, process and outcome, not whether OHS systems have been implemented and are functioning well.

References

Donabedian, A. (1988) The quality of care; how it can be assessed? *JAMA*, **260**, 1743–8.
Higashi, T., Mizoue, T., Muto, T. *et al.* (1994) Present condition of occupational health services for small-scale enterprises in Japan and their administrative support. *J. UOE.*, **16**, 309–20.
Kroon, P.J. and Overeynder, M.A. (1991) *Occupational Health Services in 6 Member States of the EC.* Amsterdam: Studiecentrum Arbeid & Gezondheid.

International Labour Organization (1985) *Proposed Recommendation Concerning Occupational Health Services*. Report of the committee on occupational health services, Provisional record. International Labour Conference, 71st session 1985, Recommendation No. 171.

JFEA (Japan Federation of Employers' Associations) (1993) *Tasks and Direction of Occupational Physicians: for the Promotion and Consolidation of Occupational Health*. JFEA (in Japanese).

JMA (Japan Medical Association) (1990) A Guideline on Certified Occupational Physicians. *Jpn J. Med. Assoc.*, **103**,1589–95 (in Japanese).

JSOH (Japan Society for Occupational Health) (1994) *A Notebook of Occupational Physician Training*. JSOH (in Japanese).

MAFF (Ministry of Agriculture, Forestry and Fisheries) (1996) *Report of Accidents Caused in the Farming Industry*. MAFF (in Japanese).

MOL (Ministry of Labour) (1994) Occupational health centers. *Occup. Hlth J.*, **17**(4), 5–9 (in Japanese).

MOL (Ministry of Labour) (1995a) Report of the study committee on the ideal method of promoting occupational health. *Occup. Hlth J.*, **18**(4), 4–7 (in Japanese).

MOL (Ministry of Labour) (1995b) *Labour Laws of Japan* 1995. The Institute of Labour Administration.

MOL (Ministry of Labour) (1996) On partial revision of Industrial Safety and Health Law. *Occup. Hlth J.*, **19**(6), 4–8 (in Japanese).

Mizoue, T., Higashi, T., Muto, T. *et al.* (1996) Activities of an occupational health organization in Japan, in special reference to services for small- and medium-scale enterprises. *Occup. Med.*, **46**, 12–16.

Muto, T., Higashi, T., Mizoue, T. *et al.* (1995a) Multiple channels for occupational health services to small-scale enterprises in Japan. *Occup. Med.*, **45**, 268–72.

Muto, T. and Fukuwatari, Y. (1995b) Relationship between companies and health insurance societies as providers of occupational health services in Japan. In: Abstracts of Quality and Audit in Occupational Health Services Conference (Glasgow).

Muto, T., Kikuchi, S., Ozawa, K. *et al.* (1995c) Barriers to health promotion in Japanese companies with special reference to health personnel. *Safety Science*, **20**, 329–34.

Muto, T., Itoh, I., Horie, S. *et al.* (1998) Roles of occupational physicians and occupational health nurses in Japan. *J. UOEH*, **20**(S), 68–73.

Okubo, T. (1994) *International Standards in Occupational Health Services*. Occupational Health Promotion Foundation (in Japanese).

Okubo, T. (1997) The present state of occupational health in Japan. *Int. Arch. Environ. Hlth*, **70**, 138–42.

Okubo, T. (1998) Recent state and future scope of occupational health in Japan. *J. Occup. Hlth*, **40**, 161–7.

Osaka Gas Co. (1990) The method of cost-containment of occupational health services. *How to Health Care*, **20**, 12–15 (in Japanese).

Rantanen, J. (1990) *Occupational Health Services: an Overview*. Geneva: World Health Organization.

SCIFOP (Study Committee on the Ideal Functions of Occupational Physicians) (1992) *Report of the Study Committee on the Ideal Functions of Occupational Physicians. Occup. Hlth J.*, **15**(4), 5–25 (in Japanese).

Takahashi, K. and Okubo, T. (1994) Current status of occupational health in Japan. *Occup. Med.*, **44**, 66–9.

Tsuchiya, K. (1991) Development of occupational health in Japan. *J. UOEH*, **13**, 191–205.

9

Government-sponsored evaluation of OHS – the Norwegian case

Terje Lie and Axel Wannag

In February 1997, the Ministry of Local Government and Labour in Norway requested an evaluation of national occupational health services (OHS) – to be completed by year-end 1998. The initial steps of this evaluation are described here. There is a discussion of how we – as evaluators – had to conceptualize the situation in order to identify the most important points to focus upon. We briefly sketch out the theories we deemed useful for the analytic part of the evaluation, and how these theories governed the data we had to collect. An account is provided of how we defined our target population and which methods we adopted for data collection. A few comments are made on preliminary findings.

Norwegian work legislation

In Norway, the employer has total responsibility for the work environment, and the health and safety of employees under the Work Environment Act, 1977. The employer is, if deemed necessary, obliged by law to recruit health and safety personnel to occupational health services (OHS). There is a duty on the part of an enterprise to obtain what is called *aid and support* to secure its work environment under the terms of the 'Provision on Safety and Health Personnel' regulation (Provision 518, 1994).

OHS themselves, however, are not legally regulated. Accordingly, no governmental agency can influence OHS directly or control their operations. In practice, however, OHS function on an open market, where they are 'the provider', and the employer is 'the purchaser'. Further, individual employers are free to organize how they obtain 'aid and support' from OHS. As a result, we see a multitude of OHS set-ups. This, in combination with the absence of quality control of service delivery, makes it reasonable to suspect that there is huge variation in the quality of the aid and support provided.

What we do know is that a fair proportion of personnel in OHS are very well trained in their profession. There are also strong indications that many employers do not exploit this potential to obtain high quality 'aid and support'. Many enterprises are accused of not being interested in providing preventive services to improve the work environment, and of prioritizing health examinations and individual health care instead. On the other hand, some employers have lately started to complain that they do not get the preventive services they want from their OHS. Overall, the situation is heterogeneous. We simply do not know what is going on.

The Norwegian government has not yet ratified the recommendations of 'Occupational Health Services for All Workers' issued by the International Labour Office (ILO, 1985). However, the Ministry of Local Government and Labour has decided to re-evaluate this position. As one of the bases for re-evaluation, the Ministry commissioned an evaluation of the present functioning of OHS as an instrument for work environment improvements – to be completed by the end of 1998.

The commission and its remit

In February 1997, the Ministry invited tenders for performance of a national OHS evaluation. It requested answers to the following questions:

- To what extent do enterprises use OHS to perform the tasks stipulated in the Work Environment Act (such as surveys and risk-evaluation of the work environment, survey and control of the health of employees in relation to work environment exposures, aid in workplace rehabilitation, documentation of advice, surveys and reports)? What are the most important and extensive activities of OHS? Is there concordance between employers' and employees' wishes and demands with regard to OHS and the tasks they prioritize?
- How are the priorities and practical work of OHS influenced by external conditions? These may be:
  (a) government laws, provisions, other regulations and actions;
  (b) other external conditions, such as the professional standards of OHS personnel and their education;
  (c) expectations and demands from employers;
  (d) expectations and demands from employees.
- To what extent are OHS established as teams including different professions? Which professions are represented and how well do they cooperate? Which profession takes which role within an OHS team? Does OHS today have the right competence (proficiency) to be able to conduct the activities specified by law?
- How important are OHS to employers and employees in the firm? Are OHS a natural and integrated part of total work-environment activities in the firm? Does cooperation between OHS personnel and employers/employees function so as to promote preventive work environment activities?
- Does the organization of OHS influence which services they provide to an enterprise? (Note that there are different organizational models:
  (a) in-house OHS departments within a firm;

    (b) OHS organized by a group of firms as a separate economic unit serving all firms in the group;

    (c) OHS set up as a private commercial enterprise owned by their own personnel;

    (d) physicians devoting a few hours a week to occupational medicine alongside their general practice;

    (e) other models of organization.)

- Do firm-related variables (such as number of employees, trade, work environment risks, others) influence the services which OHS provide to the firm?
- Do OHS lead to concrete effects being made in enterprises? Effects might include improvement in the work environment, improvement in the health of employees, and reduced sick-leave absence or other disturbances. How can any results be documented? How can the total costs and benefits of OHS – seen as an instrument for work environment improvement – be compared with alternative use of the same amount of resources for work environment improvement?

Task of the evaluators

Given the mandate from the Ministry, our task as evaluators was to transform and reformulate these questions into empirical observable measures. Figure 9.1 provides a summary of how we decided to work.

The conceptual model

Taking the Ministry mandate as a point of departure, we constructed a conceptual model capable of covering as many paragraphs in the mandate as possible within the resources allocated to us by the Ministry.

    The key starting point, both theoretically and methodologically, was to

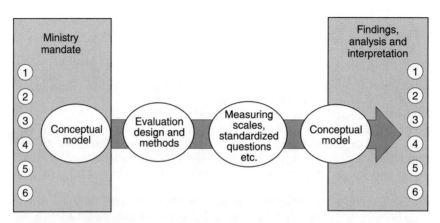

Figure 9.1 *Our work scheme*

define more precisely the targets of the project. In particular, what should be the focal points of our evaluation? The general guide provided by the Ministry, i.e. quite simply 'Evaluate OHS', was in need of elaboration.

Given the 'free market' OHS model in Norway, services depend on two parties – the company as a purchaser of services and OHS as providers. Since the employer has total responsibility for the work environment in Norway, we felt the research focus had to be revised somewhat – placing greater emphasis on the role of employers. Figure 9.2 illustrates this process in a simple model. Here, the quality of service is the outcome of interaction between company and OHS.

OHS represent professional knowledge and competence, and are expected to advise the company on matters relating to the work environment. Health personnel are responsible for the product they deliver, while the company is responsible for obtaining the necessary services and following up advice given. Accordingly, a company's ability to order the necessary services is crucial to quality, as too is its interest and motivation in monitoring and improving the work environment. This way of viewing the problem focuses on interaction between OHS and the company. We regarded such interaction as central to the functioning of an OHS organization and made it the primary focus of our attention.

Accordingly, two perspectives came to be of key importance – the company's role as purchaser and its assessment of OHS as provider; and OHS themselves, their role as provider and their judgement of the company as purchaser.

Another central factor that influences the work and effects of OHS concerns the conditions (such as negotiations, enforcement of regulations, incentives, support and so on) set by the authorities for the operation of the services provided. This aspect, however, will not be considered here.

In what follows, our intention is to describe our theoretical considerations and practical experiences in planning and initiating the evaluation. Important issues were how to collect relevant data describing the interaction between enterprises and their OHS unit, and the outcome of this interaction. Of central interest was the identification of the elements promoting or shaping such interaction.

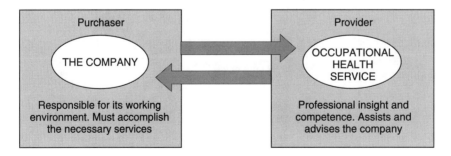

Figure 9.2 *Interaction between the enterprise and the OHS*

We chose to stick to the basic social-science tradition, which – according to Baklien (1993) – has four legs to stand on:

- 'ideal versus reality' research;
- research on effects and causality (the experimental model);
- action research;
- analysis of implementation.

Our intention was to adopt the **'ideal–reality'** perspective in analysis of the 'formal' aims and objectives of the companies, and contrast these with the actual strategies pursued. This generated a string of questions in need of operationalization:

- What are the strategic priorities of the companies?
- What services do they order from OHS personnel?
- Do they follow advice given by OHS?
- Do they invest in work-environment improvements?

From the **'cause and effect'** perspective, we wanted to analyse the results of interventions and pay-offs from companies' investments in health services. A key question here is the utility of services, seen from the point of view of both employer and employees.

Action research and **analysis of implementation** were relevant to us with regard to understanding the intervention aspect of OHS, and services when regarded as a social programme. We treated Norwegian work environment legislation, and the institutional arrangements it creates, as an ongoing programme designed to maintain and improve the work environment, and protect employees from hazardous exposures.

Our evaluation therefore, should also take into account perspectives built on other evaluation traditions, above all *programme evaluation*. Such a perspective would – in our case – bring assessment of impact and efficiency of OHS into the evaluation. Two main questions for such assessment are whether or not appropriate target groups are served, and the extent to which programme staff and management meet commitments with regard to quality and quantity of services provided (Rossi and Freeman, 1993).

Accordingly, our conceptual design came to incorporate ideas of process, structure and output (the latter seen as the distribution of

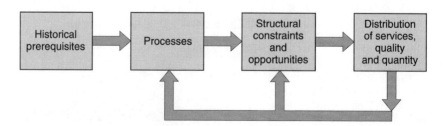

Figure 9.3 *The conceptual design*

services). The conceptual model focuses on social interaction, negotia-
tion, cooperation and decisions. Decisions, however, are always taken
with reference to constraints and opportunities, such as legal demands,
economic opportunities, attitudes, motivation and so on.

The resulting distribution of services can be interpreted in the light of
'programme' objectives (such as legal demands). Experiences and learning might feed back both on the process itself (e.g. the need for better
communication), and on structural constraints (e.g. the need for better
legislation or incentives).

Study population – companies and their OHS units

Central to any evaluation is identification and sampling of the right
population to study. Accordingly, we had to find a way of sampling
correctly from the 'universe' of all Norwegian OHS and their corre-
sponding enterprises. But trying to start with a sample of OHS units
immediately led us into difficulties. There were no authoritative records
of the services, even though some 'informal' registers exist. Using such
registers might have resulted in a biased sample of both services and
companies.

We chose to adopt the opposite approach. We sampled companies
first, and then looked up the OHS they used. An operative register of
companies was obtained from Statistics Norway. From this register, we
were able to draw a random sample of companies (limited to those
obliged to purchase OHS), stratified by size and geographic location.

We had to consider that a majority of companies in the sample would
have an OHS unit of their own, but that some (especially small companies) would not. In our sampling model, we assumed a certain coverage
of OHS among companies (dependent on size), and a response rate of
about 65%. We decided to sample 1000 companies from the Statistics
Norway register, based on this model. We expected the number of OHS
units to be slightly less than the number of companies, since one single
unit might cover several companies. In the end, we obtained a sample of
251 companies with an agreement with an OHS organization, plus a list
of the health services they used.

Data collection

Given our focus on interaction – and the outcome of this – we selected
the following methods of data collection:

A sample survey

This took the form of a quantitative enquiry based on questionnaires sent
by post to companies, safety deputies (required by law in Norway, and
elected by employees) and OHS units. Thus, as sketched out in Figure
9.4, we judged OHS from three angles – the manager of the company,
the safety deputy in the company and the occupational health service.

We developed three questionnaires, one for each party, but with quite

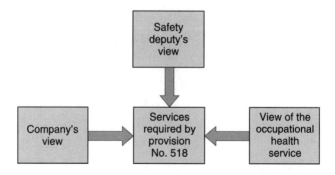

Figure 9.4 *Triangulation of survey data: parties included in the evaluation of the OHS*

similar item structures. The version sent to OHS, however, contained specific questions relating to organization and resources, and the companies they served. Companies were posed additional questions, related to their work environment and OHS received. Safety deputies received a similar questionnaire, but one phrased from the point of view of employees.

The construction of questionnaires takes time (Mordal, 1989), and we revised ours several times. Given our focus on interaction between the parties, we were particularly eager to find formulations and themes that reflected the procedural nature of this interaction. One way of measuring this is to let the parties involved take a stand on several statements describing the relation between the company and its OHS. We devised 24 such statements, to which each respondent could agree or disagree. The statements describe, for example, the quality of cooperation, the competence of the company to order services, the interest of the company in the work of OHS personnel, and so on. From these statements, we were later able to construct relevant indexes based on the empirical data obtained.

Other items in the questionnaires covered:

- the company's task priorities in relation to the work environment;
- the tasks being accomplished by OHS for the company;
- the company's priorities in relation to its needs;
- consequences of efforts and actions in the work environment on areas such as sick leave, accidents, injuries, work-related illness, company finances etc;
- investments designed to improve the work environment.

In Figure 9.5 we show an example of how we constructed a particular question (one that appears in all the questionnaires). In this item, we seek out the priorities of the company on different work environment issues, and ask to what degree OHS had assisted the company on these issues.

Tasks	The priorities of the company			Who assists the company?		Not of immediate importance
	High	Medium	Low	OHS	Others	
A Registration and assessment of physical, chemical, and biological exposures in the company	☐	☐	☐	☐	☐	☐
B Registration and assessment of the employees' degree of control over work	☐	☐	☐	☐	☐	☐
C Proposals for preventative actions	☐	☐	☐	☐	☐	☐
D Monitoring the health status of the employees	☐	☐	☐	☐	☐	☐

Figure 9.5 *Example from the questionnaire: questions mapping the priorities of the enterprise*

A case study

Ten companies were drawn at random from the register maintained by Statistics Norway. In the sampling procedure, we chose three geographic regions, reflecting both urban and non-urban areas. The target population was the same as for the quantitative enquiry, i.e. Norwegian companies obliged to maintain OHS.

This part of the study was designed as a qualitative enquiry, for which evaluators personally interviewed representatives of the company, safety deputies and representatives of the OHS. Item coverage was much the same as for the sample survey, but personal contact made in-depth information possible (Wadel, 1996). The case study was used to provide an additional source of information on the basis of which the quantitative study could be validated in general terms.

The interviews took place either in groups with all three parties present, or with each party separately.

Data collected

Status of data collection in August 1998 was as follows. Following one reminder, the company response rate was 70% ($n = 256$), the OHS response rate 77% ($n = 281$), and the safety deputy response rate 70% ($n = 219$). Responses from all three parties constituted 50% of the material, and those from two parties 43%. The remainder are single responses from either the company, OHS personnel, or the employees' safety deputy.

We regard the number of responses to be large enough to make generalizations based on the data. Responses are non-skewed with regard to parameters such as company size and geographic location.

Experiences so far

Identification of enterprises with OHS

To obtain information on whether an enterprise had an OHS unit or not, and also where it was located (name, address, telephone number), we mailed a small folder to all enterprises in our sample. The folder had a 'tear-off' pre-stamped section on which the enterprise should provide information before mailing it back to us.

Among returns (511 out of 920), 75% reported affiliation to an OHS unit. The number of returns indicated that companies without OHS affiliation did not reply, which could lead to bias in our sample. We were, however, able to control for geographic location, size and industry. In these respects, our sample was found to be unbiased.

Some information from enterprises was not reconcilable with information obtained from OHS. Some OHS units did not recognize the enterprise that had claimed to be their service recipient. Following sorting of the sample population in the light of additional information, we ended up with a sample of 365 enterprises.

The enterprise and OHS database

We made our database in Access, using information on both enterprises and OHS units, and updated it whenever new data arrived. The database also contains very useful information from Statistics Norway, which enabled us to check – among other things – on possible sample biases.

The questionnaire

We received rather few telephone calls from respondents to the questionnaire. Larger enterprises, with a variety of different units, sometimes called to discuss which unit they should give information about. To us, it seemed that it was not at all clear to the enterprise which of their departments bore the legal responsibility to engage OHS.

The OHS units that called were more concerned about specific formulations and exact meanings in the questionnaire. This is relevant to the problem of survey validity and reliability.

Validity and reliability of an evaluation instrument are central to all empirical evaluation work, and considerable attention has been devoted to them in the scientific literature. In this context, we should simply like to draw attention to Galtung's (1967) view that 'validity' is, to a large extent, an epistemological question, and not just one of measurement. By contrast, reliability can, at least to some degree, be checked using statistical techniques.

It is premature to draw conclusions concerning the validity and reliability of our data, but we have already received some indications. Missing responses, for example, might indicate that respondents did not understand a question, or that – for various reasons – a question was difficult to answer. In our data, however, the missing-response rate is low, seldom exceeding 4% on any one single item.

But some questions do not seem to have functioned as well as we hoped. Among those shown in Figure 9.5, the question on priorities was easily understood. But the question 'Who assists the company?' led to some misunderstandings. The matrix we used for this item – with several questions demanding much information – might be difficult for respondents, and may have resulted in reduced data quality.

Questions that require a lot of knowledge and documented information that is not easily accessible are difficult to answer. An example from our questionnaire is the item on the effects of sick leave on an enterprise's investment in work-environment improvement. Both the enterprise and the OHS need to have some idea of the effect, but how much this reflects fiction and how much fact is difficult to assess.

Strangely, the question to OHS on their number of personnel in different professions was sometimes difficult to answer, and clarification had to be obtained through telephone contents.

The items built on a combination of structured and open questions have proved useful. The additional information given in open-comment sections was often very instructive.

Data analysis

We have used the SPSS package, and keep three separate files for each category of respondents. We are able to merge data from the three files for the simultaneous study of responses from all three sets of respondents (triangulation).

Reliability

We have applied SPSS reliability tests to relevant items to obtain some preliminary views on reliability. On our attitudinal questions, we have obtained an alpha value of 0.70, which is regarded as quite high.

Preliminary findings

We will use the index 'visible occupational service' as an example. The index is composed of several items, such as 'inspire the company', 'market competence', 'inform about work environment', and so on. About 50% of managers in the companies agree with these statements. At about 75%, OHS professionals tend to agree more strongly than managers, while employees' safety deputies score between the two (at about 60%).

A *t*-test (in this case, we used the paired-sample test), measuring the differences between the mean scores of the parties, has demonstrated statistically significant differences. The parties do not agree with each other. This means that managers, OHS personnel and safety deputies judge the visibility of OHS differently, even within the same companies.

Employees' safety deputies, in their comments, are most inclined to point to lack of visibility and access to OHS as the most important issue for employees. One does not even know who OHS personnel are: 'What service?' a deputy asks. Another writes, 'They [OHS personnel] should be more visible to employees. Who are they?' A manager writes, 'The occupational health service does not visit our company. This is perhaps due to the fact that we are a small company. They have promised to come, but nothing happens.'

Both the statistics and the verbal comments illustrate some of the expectations that company managers and safety deputies have of OHS. Judging from the data gathered, OHS professionals believe themselves to be more visible and accessible than they are perceived to be by the other parties. Obviously, there is a mismatch between expectations of clients and services provided.

From our evaluation perspective, all parties should share the responsibility to correct this situation. Managers need to adopt a more active attitude towards OHS, and be more specific in their claims and orders. OHS professionals should foster relations with their companies, provide better information on how they work, and – if necessary – explain why certain expectations cannot be met.

References

Baklien, B. (1993) Evalueringsforskning i Norge. *Tidsskr. Samfunnsforskning* [*Journal of Social Research*], **3**, 275–280.

Galtung, J. (1967) *Theory and Methods of Social Research.* Oslo: Universitetsforlaget.

International Labour Office (1985) *Occupational Health Services*: Report IV (1)/1985, 71 session. Geneva: ILO.

Labour Inspectorate (1994) *Provision of the 'Work Environment Act' on Safety and Health Personnel* (no. 518), Oslo: Ministry of Local Government and Labour.

Ministry of Local Government and Labour (1977) *Act Relating to Worker Protection and Working Environment* ('Work Environment Act'). Oslo: Grøndahl Dreyer.

Mordal, T. (1989) *'Som man spør får man svar'* ['Ask a stupid question, get a stupid answer']: *Arbeid med survey-opplegg.* Oslo: Tano.

Rossi, P.H. and Howard, E.F. (1993) *Evaluation: A Systematic Approach.* Newbury Park, CA: Sage Publications.

Wadel, C. (1996) *Humanistisk sosiologi.* Bergen: Fagbokforlaget.

Note: The survey providing the basis for this chapter's text has been published as a report with bibliographical reference identity:

Lie, T. (1999) Evaluering av verne – og helsepersonale i virksomhetene. (Evaluation of occupational health services in Norway). (Forfatter: Terje Lie, Jan Erik Karlsen og Joren Elise Tharaldsen.) Stavanger: Rogalandforskning, 1999–XII, 160 + 10 + 27s; 30 cm (Rogalandforskning, RF; 1999/007). ISBN 82-7220-963-2.

10

Internal and external evaluation of OHS – the German case

Karl Kuhn

The current state of and recent developments in occupational health services (OHS) in Germany is surveyed. Emphasis is placed on the diversity of working life with regard to industrial sectors and size of enterprise. The account centres on statutory obligations with regard to occupational safety and health imposed on German employers and their various responses to these. Small and medium-sized enterprises require special attention. Organizational models of care, quality assurance approaches, outcome monitoring, preventive medical examinations, risk evaluation and care specifications are discussed. Documentation and statistics have a key role to play. Diversity demands a broad range of care solutions.

In 1997, some 82 million people lived in the Federal Republic of Germany. The population steadily increased from 1991 to 1997 – by 2.2 million – as a result of immigration. By contrast, the number of people in work in Germany fell between 1991 and 1997 – by 1.6 million, from 37.4 million to 35.8 million. The number of companies with employees liable to make social insurance contributions (enterprises with at least one employee) had risen to 2023 million by 1997. The crucial factor in this increase was the continuing growth in the number of small enterprises with up to 5 employees – to 1361 million in 1997. By contrast, the number of medium and large enterprises decreased, the number of firms with more than 500 employees fell to 5035 in 1997.

The largest growth in companies took place in the service sector. Here, the number of companies had risen to 731 834 by 1997. The opposite trend was observed in the agricultural, forestry and fisheries sector. And in manufacturing the number of generally large firms continued to fall – to 334 534 in 1997. In the same year, the number of companies in the construction industry was 192 612 and in the trading sector, 427 452.

The large number of companies and their wide distributions across sectors and by size mean that a host of different care models are required to allow for diverse organizational circumstances.

Basic obligations of employers

Under new legislation in Germany, the employer has far-reaching responsibilities for the safety and health of company employees. But the Occupational Safety and Health Act (ASiG) clearly states that employers may commission reliable and expert people to fulfil the obligations that they have to satisfy by law. In particular, the ASiG lays down a variety of basic obligations. Here are just some of them:

- An employer must provide a suitable occupational safety and health organization and the staff it requires.
- Occupational safety and health measures must be integrated and observed at all company levels.
- The employer must evaluate work conditions within the company, and take protective action in line with the risk potential established.
- The employer has to check protective measures for effectiveness and, where necessary, tailor them to new developments and changing know-how. That is, *there is a basic obligation to perform an internal evaluation of risks and measures implemented.*
- The employer must document the results of risk evaluation and protective measures taken (so-called 'documentation').
- The employer must inform the works and staff councils about all measures relating to occupational safety and health at the company.
- According to Section 5 of the ASiG, the employer is obliged to appoint 'experts for occupational safety and health' to look after employees' safety. OHS experts can be appointed full-time or on a temporary basis. They can be employed by the company, work on a freelance basis, or even belong to an external service commissioned by the company for care and consultancy (under Section 19 of the ASiG).
- According to Section 2 of the ASiG, the employer has to appoint or commission works physicians to provide medical care for employees. These physicians can be appointed as full-time or temporary staff. They can be employed by the company, work on a freelance basis, or even belong to an external service charged by the company to perform the work.

Models of workplace medical care

Given the sectoral diversity of German industry and the large number and kinds of companies involved, a wide range of models have been developed for the implementation of statutory provisions. Large companies generally satisfy requirements by means of in-house prevention services, whereas small and medium enterprises usually have to buy OHS from outside.

The opportunities for small enterprises to provide medical care are as follows:

- Engage a full-time works physician from a large company who looks after group companies as part of his/her regular work as well as outside firms on behalf of the company.

- Set up a works physician centre – possibly a centre sponsored by an accident insurance company, an independent centre (regional, national), or a centre sponsored by an organization.
- Engage an occupational physician with his/her own practice – working alone, working in a practice for occupational medicine, or working in a joint practice with a panel doctor.
- Engage a part-time works physician – a full-time panel/contract doctor, a full-time hospital doctor, full-time doctor at a government authority or in administration, or a full-time works physician at a major company (with permission to work part-time).

The situation is similar for OHS experts. They may work in similar organizational constellations, but also have to meet certain requirements with regard to expertise. Description of these requirements in detail would go beyond the scope of this chapter.

To choose from among these options, employers should make an assessment of demand based on the accident-prevention regulations, obtain quotations, check value for money with a critical eye, and then order the services or conclude a contract. A key part of this contract should be company-specific, containing specifications geared to prevention and covering the services to be provided. Note also that the legislation stipulates that companies must ensure continual improvement in occupational safety and health.

The statutory requirements are designed to achieve a high standard of occupational safety and health in the workplace. However, it should be obvious, given the huge scale of the prevention market, that an overall high level of OHS cannot be guaranteed. Deficiencies in care may relate to numerous aspects of prevention services – inadequate qualifications, low-priced suppliers with poor services, no or inadequate consulting on workplace design, exclusion of important fields of action (e.g. psychosocial stresses), inadequate efficiency reviews, no consultancy to suit specific needs, and so on. One major problem lies in the calculation of deployment times. Generally, they do not permit a comprehensive range of OHS, and company health care is therefore limited to 'medical examinations'.

A recent representative survey of 11 800 selected enterprises established the following with regard to the perceived significance of occupational safety and health:

- At major companies, occupational safety and health is, in two cases out of three, an integral part of mission statements and management principles, or is regarded as an 'unwritten law'.
- At companies with 50–250 employees, under half adopt such a favourable stance.
- At small enterprises, by contrast, there is often no time for such formalities.

However, such enterprises tend to be aware that occupational safety and health plays an important role in relation to atmosphere at work. Every third enterprise expressed this view. Over 40% of small enterprises (with fewer than 10 employees) criticized the statutory provisions on the grounds that they were far too complicated. In a survey of employees, 10% thought that their employer did not bother about occupational safety and health. In sum, the smaller the enterprise, the lower is the significance of and interest in occupational safety and health.

Quality assurance

Questions of how the quality of workplace care can be ensured by external and internal OHS are becoming more important. Here, too, Germany has taken account of a wide variety of possibilities:

- Integration of occupational safety and health into company quality assurance systems.
- Occupational safety and health management systems, such as the ASCA (Health and Safety Check in Installations) in Hesse. ASCA operates within a concept of integrated maintenance of health and safety standards, summarizing and pursuing all relevant aspects of the medical, social and technical industrial health and safety standards, employee-adjusted work design and labour organization.The starting point is a systems analysis designed not only to reveal deficiencies in occupational safety and health but also to analyse interaction between company workflows and functions.
- Large external services with certified quality assurance and quality management systems. Examples include BAD (the employers' liability-insurance and occupational health service), which employs 1500 works physicians and OHS experts. BAD looks after 17 000 companies in Germany through its 20 regional branches and 175 centres, and is certified to DIN EN ISO-9001.
- Voluntary quality groups. One of these has been established by Germany's largest association for industrial care, and the Association of Works Physicians will adopt the same approach. To this end, it has founded its own company for quality in occupational safety and health (GQA). Its expert advisory council includes the Federal Minister of Labour and Social Affairs, and management and workers' representatives. After positive conclusion of a preliminary investigation, GQA submits to the service provider a quotation for inspection of the staff, material and organizational quality of its safety service. The basis for the quality review is a checklist confirmed by the expert advisory council.
- The Federal Working Group of External Occupational Health Services (BAGA) has developed binding quality criteria for its members in order to ensure high quality of OHS. These quality criteria relate to organizational and staff requirements, to the structuring of contracts with the employer, and to the performance of tasks (scope and documentation of the services).
- Services without quality assurance.

Monitoring of output

Key statistics at both state and company level constitute an important resource for the monitoring and evaluation of the development of occupational safety and health. Also, the new legislation has extended the reporting obligation of the federal government in the occupational safety and health arena. For example, the ASiG states the following:

> The federal government shall submit to the German Bundestag and Bundesrat every year by 31 December of the year following the year under review a statistical report on the situation of occupational safety and health and on the accident and occupational-disease figures for the Federal Republic of Germany. This report shall summarize the reports of the accident insurance companies and the annual reports of the regional authorities responsible for occupational safety and health. Every four years the report shall contain a comprehensive review of the development of industrial accidents and occupational diseases, their costs and the occupational safety and health action taken.

State monitoring of safety and health represents a rough evaluation instrument for checking developments in safety and health, and in morbidity, mortality and early-retirement parameters (in longitudinal cross-section). An important element, and major factor, is the cost trend in the prevention sector, and also the financial balance of activities in the occupational safety and health arena.

The most recent draft report indicates a favourable economic balance from a sociopolitical viewpoint, since the number of industrial accidents in Germany fell from 2.7 million in 1960 to 1.6 million in 1997. This decline is not least remarkable because, over the same period, there was an increase in the number of full-time workers from 24.9 to 38.1 million. The number of accidents per 1000 full-time workers fell from 109 to 42 during the period, meaning that the accident rate has dropped to its lowest level since the foundation of the Federal Republic of Germany.

As a result of this favourable trend, the share of accident insurance contributions in the social insurance budget fell from 2.2% to 1.5% over the past decades, despite substantial cost increases for pensions and rehabilitation. Whereas in 1960 companies had to spend DM1.51 per DM100 in wages, in 1997 this figure was only DM 1.40. Accident insurance is the only branch in the German social insurance system that exhibits stable, even slightly declining, contributions over many years. This can be interpreted as a positive long-term outcome for occupational safety and health care.

Increasing importance is also being attached to occupational safety and health indicators at company level. Accident rates and occupational illness figures have always been very important for German companies because accident-insurance contributions are linked (for better or for worse) to the level of industrial accidents. Industrial accidents increase contributions, and prevention therefore takes on great significance. At the same time, absenteeism figures, which are made available by health insurance funds for each company, sector and even professional group, are becoming increasingly important. These statistics provide a company with an indication of whether it has a higher or lower absenteeism rate than the sector and regional averages.

Further comparisons are possible because data on employees unable to work can be broken down by age, sex, profession, diagnosis, and so on within a company, and thereby furnish the company with information on which areas are critical and where preventive action has to be taken. This information can be expressed in monetary terms, and increase pressure on external services to take action. The success of OHS can be measured directly from trends in these key statistics.

Since absenteeism rates have now become important for safeguarding locations and capital expenditure, the significance of these key figures has risen tremendously in recent years. Statutory health insurance funds now offer standardized questionnaires to survey disruptions to well-being, perceived stresses, the working climate, leadership style, suggestions for improvement, and so on. The results of the surveys are used by the health insurance funds, and are usually also made available to the company together with data on absenteeism and the results of health circles (in the form of health reports).

The company, sector or guild thereby obtains a fairly accurate picture of the health situation, and a company can directly present its prevention service with this information. As a result, OHS are put under pressure to achieve success. Since services are expensive, the company is confronted with the question of what all the efforts – such as medical check-ups, risk assessments, safety rounds, and so on – achieve if the absenteeism rate remains high. The figures are regarded as a measure of efficiency.

In many sectors of the economy, such as the automobile industry, key figures on absenteeism and accident rates are employed for the benchmarking of suppliers. This compels suppliers to raise occupational safety and health in their companies to a high level.

Preventive medical examinations

To permit companies to adopt special preventive measures as instruments of secondary prevention, statutory accident insurance funds (including the Berufsgenossenschaft) have issued principles for preventive medical examinations. Since 1974, an obligation to perform such examinations has been laid down in law. Principles of prevention have been formulated for 44 hazardous or stressful activities (so far), providing a foundation for as uniform a check-up procedure as possible, and also as standardized an evaluation as possible of surveys of examination findings. Altogether, 47 different preventive medical examinations have so far been established (due to the fact that some principles are subdivided). Principles for the examinations are drawn up according to latest scientific expertise, which is recognized both nationally and internationally. Continual adaption to new occupational health and scientific expertise and new statutory provisions relating to occupational safety and health have resulted in the number of principles steadily increasing in recent years.

As part of a study by the Federal Institute for Occupational Safety and Health, the total number of all examinations conducted in accordance with these principles was plotted as a function of time. Preventive medical examinations between 1979 and 1995 – a total of 38.5 million check-ups – were recorded. Examination results are divided into four categories:

- No health reservations;
- No health reservations under certain preconditions;
- Limited health reservations;
- Persistent health reservations.

More than 4 million examinations are now conducted each year in Germany. It has been shown that the two groups where limited or persistent health reservations were held remained almost unchanged at a constantly low figure. The number of examinations with the result 'No health reservations under certain preconditions' showed a slight overall increase in the survey period, while 'No health reservations' rose fourfold over the same period.

The results give rise to the question of whether, on analysis of these figures, a preventive effect is being achieved for the individual. The analysis showed that in 1995 'Health reservations' were expressed in the medical examinations of over 14% of all workers. Without going into further details of individual health complaints, this result underlines the preventive medical significance of the examinations according to the principles developed. Nevertheless, taking a critical view, it should be mentioned that – in addition to a reduction in the number of examinations – there should be an intensification of individual examinations so as to achieve an improvement in the quality of preventive action.

It is also established that the medico-epidemiological benefit of preventive medical examinations needs to be optimized. Improved documentation of health data is regarded as an important contribution towards this. Such basic documentation should also provide information regarding the extent to which health complaints observed are attributable to workplace-associated risks. On the basis of comprehensive documentation, a risk-adapted, individual health prevention scheme for employees can be successful and, in the future, economically justifiable.

Risk evaluation

The new occupational safety and health legislation obliges the employer to conduct an evaluation of risks to employees at work, and also to determine what occupational safety and health measures are required. Risk evaluation means the detection and assessment of possible causes of accidents and health disorders as a result of work activities. Its aim is to derive measures to eliminate risks. The following questions should be evaluated:

- What risks can arise?
- Which people are affected by the risks?
- Are conditions in the workplace acceptable and – in particular – do they comply with rules and regulations, codes of practice, the state of the art, and the performance qualifications of employees?
- Are improvements possible?
- What sort of measures are required and how urgently?

- What requirements do planned occupational safety and health measures, new work stations, new work equipment and new work procedures have to meet?

These risk factors relate to all employment sectors.

In Germany, there is a great need in companies (especially in small and medium-sized enterprises) for support in the implementation of risk evaluation. All OHS institutions have now developed instruments offering possible assistance. Some of these are sector-specific, others stress-oriented, still others workplace-oriented. Alternatively, they are aimed explicitly at the experts who perform the work. As the results have to be documented, there is an opportunity to conduct risk evaluation at a high level, and also to put pressure on prevention-service providers to offer appropriate quality when an instrument is deployed.

Evaluations of some branch organizations are now available. For example, assessments were conducted by the Berufsgenossenschaft at roughly 25 000 companies with fewer than 31 employees in the metal industry. About 50 doctors from 24 works/company physician centres and about 65 technical supervisors of the Berufsgenossenschaft were involved in this campaign. Reports for companies were prepared during site visits, and the need for action to improve safety and occupational health determined. The reports make up an important element in the documentation of results of risk evaluations and in the occupational safety and health measures established. The company must keep this documentation in accordance with Section 6 of the ASiG.

One advantage of this procedure is that relevant data obtained from surveys of all small enterprises can be recorded and processed to develop preventive action for specific target groups. Moreover, sector-specific stress profiles can be drawn up on the basis of the data obtained. Action plans have been prepared for use at small enterprises in cooperation with the Berufsgenossenschaft, guilds, health insurance funds, journeyman committees and the authorities responsible.

Specifications

As with risk evaluation, numerous OHS organizations now perform their tasks on the basis of 'specifications for occupational safety and/or health care', which are established for the sector in question. These specifications are broken down under the following headings:

- Risk characterization;
- Risk assessment;
- Establishment of safety and health objectives and measures;
- Documentation on risk assessment and safety and health measures;
- Breakdown of deployment times according to focal tasks.

With the aid of these specifications, which can be modified in consultation with the company in question, recognized shortcomings can be tackled and eliminated. As a result, the company is put in a position to recognize the need for action and help to comply with the statutory provisions. As far as pricing is concerned, variations between sectors, company sizes and individual needs for care are generally taken into account.

Concluding remarks

The large number of companies in Germany demands a host of care possibilities. As a rule, procedures that permit internal and external evaluation are specified for providing the service. Nevertheless, numerous small enterprises have previously not had adequate care. A large number of on-going projects have been embarked upon in an attempt to develop effective and efficient solutions.

Bibliography

Maschinenbau und Metallberufsgenossenschaft (1998) *Arbeitsbedingte Gesundheitsgefahren in Kleinbetrieben der Metallbearbeitung und -verarbeitung.* (Work related hazards in SMEs in the manufacture of basic metals.) Dusseldorf: MetallBG.

Weihrauch, M., Lehnert, G., Valentin, H. and Welte, D. (1998) *Entwicklung und derzeitiger Stand arbeitsmedizinischer Vorsorgeuntersuchungen nach berufsgenossenschaftlichen Grundsätzen* (Development and the present state of occupational health check-ups according to guidelines of the Berufsgenossenschaften). Bremerhaven: Wirtschaftsverlag NW.

11

Data-based outcome evaluation of an occupational health programme – the US case

Michael Weaver, Kathleen Brown and Jim Hilyer

Despite being an important part of overall programme evaluation, process evaluation does not access the pieces of information needed for programme planning and assessment of effectiveness. Evaluation of programme outcomes – in terms of both current status and future goals – is critical for identification of a population's occupational health needs and assessment of a programme's effectiveness. This chapter describes components of a successful comprehensive occupational health and safety programme. Information is provided on utilizing outcomes – the major evaluative mechanism for cost containment in the case study presented – for data-based programme planning and evaluation. The issue of incentives for participation is also discussed.

Soaring costs for health of staff

Over the past 10 years, soaring medical costs for employee health in the USA have challenged companies to evaluate expenses and attempt to control costs. The situation is alarming, with total national medical expenses of $949 billion in 1994, 55–80% of which are borne by employees (Kizer, *et al.*, 1995; HCFA, 1996). Annual medical expenditures have been escalating at such at pace that some companies have experienced increases of up to 20% per year. Such increases have prompted American companies to implement programmatic and evaluative strategies to contain employee costs.

Components of an occupational health and safety programme

In the early years of company health and safety programmes, employers were largely concerned with providing on-site first aid and safety training. As programmes have evolved to provide for worker health and safety, and also cover medical costs, the range of programme components has expanded. Included in current comprehensive efforts are: identification of employee health risks; careful design of medical-benefit plans; job analyses, hazard assessments and safety training; physical-fitness facilities, including fitness testing and training; targeted programmes to modify physical and mental health risks; and provision of treatment for the ill and injured.

Health promotion or wellness programmes have been developed to identify employees at risk of heart disease, cancer and injury. Early identification of health risks and intervention in relation to disease aim to minimize the catastrophic costs associated with acute major illness. Over the past two decades, companies have initiated programmes of this kind to encourage their employees to adopt healthier lifestyles. Companies have developed no-smoking policies, offered more nutritious food selections in work site cafeterias and vending machines, and provided a culture that promotes wellness. The work site is considered an ideal location for health promotion – due to peer support, convenience, and opportunities for long-term intervention.

A further component of a comprehensive occupational health and safety programme involves design of a medical benefits package to ensure cost-efficient, quality primary care. Typically, employers provide several options for medical benefit or health insurance plans. The plans offered by health maintenance organizations (HMOs), which provide a primary-care gatekeeper and full coverage for routine physical examinations, are generally preferred by employers due to their capacity to control medical costs. Employers go into partnership with insurers to structure these plans so that monthly employee contributions, co-payments and deductibles are lower, thereby encouraging employees to select the preferred plans. Companies can form alliances to influence insurers to offer medical benefits plans that emphasize health and medical cost control. In meetings with insurers, employers can exert the leverage provided by the potential for a large subscriber group to mandate the formation of limited provider networks and the development of interventions that address specific employee health risks.

To reduce injury incidence and costs, safety initiatives encompass a full spectrum of assessment and training within a comprehensive occupational health programme. Job analyses and hazard assessments are conducted to identify situations that may result in injuries. Rather than focusing on employee training as a means of injury prevention, a comprehensive programme emphasizes identification of job-related physical performance requirements, job hazards, state of the art protective equipment, and work redesign as ways of decreasing injuries. Data are collected and analysed to identify job-related physical performance levels and patterns of injuries and costs. Utilizing these data, safety programmes are evaluated, and improvements are made to ensure a safe workplace.

Many companies now offer physical fitness facilities, fitness trails and discounted memberships of private-exercise clubs as strategies to encourage employee participation in physical activity. Recognizing that physical fitness protects workers from injury, fitness evaluations of employees in high-risk occupations are conducted on a regular basis. Companies procure equipment, and staff facilities with fitness professionals who can design programmes that attract employees. In addition, programmes for strengthening, conditioning, and rehabilitating injured workers can also be conducted within a company fitness centre.

The final component of comprehensive occupational health and safety programmes encompasses programmes designed to prevent and treat specific conditions. For example, employee assistance programmes, usually contracted with an outside vendor, offer employees confidential mental health counselling and treatment on an outpatient basis. Company occupational health clinics also provide early treatment for injuries, and reduce the costs attributable to hospital emergency visits and lost time.

Why evaluate outcomes?

Process-based evaluation of programmes run by occupational health services (OHS) provides information about programme function. Although an important part of programme evaluation, process evaluation does not access the pieces of information needed for programme planning and assessment of effectiveness. An evaluation of programme outcomes – both in terms of current status and in relation to future goals – is critical for identification of a population's occupational health needs and evaluation of programme effectiveness.

As a first step in the outcome-evaluation process, the programme team needs to identify and prioritize occupational health outcomes of importance to the target population. Ideally, the outcomes selected should:

• be empirically based;
• reflect important health issues in terms of morbidity, mortality, and/ or cost within the target population;
• be amenable to modification using a worksite-based approach.

Sources of empirical information for decision-making are both external and internal. External sources may include research literature and industry and/or government publications, such as statistics, standards, or goals. Internal sources include data collected directly from the target population, and may also encompass information from health screenings, HMOs and occupational injury reports.

A municipal example: the City of Birmingham, Alabama

Beginning in 1984, the City of Birmingham, Alabama initiated multiple strategies to control escalating medical costs. With costs rising approximately 19% per year, there was a need for cost containment of medical benefits (Harvey et al., 1993; Brown et al., 1995). The strategies developed included an all-employee wellness programme, health-insurance options limited to HMOs, stronger safety programming, a fitness facility, mandatory physical activity programmes, fitness evaluations, integration of a pre-existing employee-assistance programme, and a dedicated occupational medicine clinic for care of injured employees. An over 55% reduction in annual hospital days and a 57% reduction in forecast costs were achieved. Annual injuries and injury costs were reduced by 10% among public safety workers, who were required to participate in mandatory fitness programmes and testing (Hilyer and Artz, 1992). Medical insurance costs have remained stable in relation to payroll (3.8% in 1975, 11.6% in 1985 and 11.2% in 1995) and benefits budget (16.3% in 1975, 40.2% in 1985, and 40.9% in 1995). As a result of performance in relation to these and other outcome measures, the Good Health Programme has been awarded national recognition. It obtained the C. Everett Koop Award in 1993, the Exemplary Public Worksite Health Promotion Award of the National Association for Public Worksite Health Promotion in 1994, and the Best Practice Organization designation of the International Benchmarking Clearinghouse in 1995.

The City of Birmingham Occupational Safety and Health 'Working Well' programme comprises an extensive network (see Box 11.1). The Director of the Personnel Department and Director of Occupational Safety and Health oversee the components of the programme. The University of Alabama School of Nursing at Birmingham manages the wellness programme, and also a back school and a medical-services clinic.

Box 11.1 City of Birmingham Working Well components

- Health screening and health-risk appraisals
- Health promotion
- Health maintenance organization plans for prepaid medical services
- Hazard analysis and safety inspections
- Safety promotion and training
- Physical fitness facility
- Fitness testing
- Job task evaluations
- Fitness programmes
- Rehabilitation programmes
- Back school for back-injured workers
- Employee assistance for personal problems
- 24-hour employee assistance hot line
- Occupational medical services clinic
- Injury care and work-related medical examinations
- Early return to work and case management

The Good Health Programme is designed to enhance the health and safety of City of Birmingham employees through the implementation of programmes targeting selected general and occupational-specific health-risk factors. Ultimately, it is expected that control or reduction of these risks will:

- reduce the prevalence of the selected risk factors;
- reduce the incidence of occupational injuries;
- reduce expenditures for occupational injury treatment;
- reduce expenditures for non-occupational health problems;
- reduce lost productivity related to both occupational and non-occupational health problems.

While the Good Health Programme contains elements peculiar to governmental units, the general structure of outcome identification and evaluation can be generalized to all occupational health service programmes. Most of the specific outcomes addressed are also generically applicable to the work site.

Benefits of data-based service planning

Programming for the City of Birmingham has required strategic planning and cooperation between the Personnel Department and occupational safety and health professionals. Integral to the success of the cost-containment effort is the evaluation of multiple components of the programme. An early goal was to develop an integrated database that would include information on health risks, medical claims, absenteeism, injuries, injury costs, and physical performance. Evaluation was incorporated into the project at the beginning stages of planning, and most discussions of programmes now have a data-based reference point.

The database is utilized for evaluation of the outcomes of the various components of the programme, and is beneficial for identifying trends and groups of employees that require targeted interventions. From these data, the City of Birmingham Personnel Department, insurers and occupational safety and health professionals, can identify and discuss the top ten medical costs and top ten injuries, and trends in health risks. They can also compare these data with national goals. Individual reports of health risks over the past five years are prepared for each employee participating in the health-risk appraisals, and then distributed to them in confidential sealed envelopes. Employees are counselled at health screenings when their individual reports indicate a need for change in their health risks.

Utilization of outcome measures

Both national and Alabama health statistics provided a starting point for determining which general health risk factors to address within the Good Health Programme (US Department of Health and Human Resources, 1991; Alabama Department of Public Health, 1994). Levels of risk for cardiovascular disease were regarded as outcome measures of primary importance (see Box 11. 2 for these and other primary outcome measures) – given their prevalence, costs of care, impact on risk with regard to other disease entities (e.g. cancer), and relationships to lost productivity (Forrester et al., 1996; Weaver et al., 1998). In addition, accepted behavioural and medical interventions – to impact significantly on morbidity and mortality from heart disease – are available and amenable to work site implementation. Exercise, cigarette smoking, body composition, blood pressure, resting heart rate, diet, and serum lipid levels were all identified as cardiovascular disease health-risk outcomes to target for intervention and evaluation. The outcome measures are evaluated biennially in non-public safety employees.

Standards for specific high-risk occupations (e.g. those of the Fire Service Joint Labor Management Wellness/Fitness Initiative Task Force,

1997) were used to identify the occupation-specific functional status outcome measures to target. These measures included pulmonary function, hearing (firefighters only, due to occupational exposure to high levels of noise, fumes and particulates), muscle strength, aerobic fitness and flexibility. Public safety workers (police and fire department employees), due to the demands of their jobs, are evaluated annually. Additionally, prior to institution of a hepatitis B vaccination programme

Box 11.2 City of Birmingham primary outcome evaluation measures

- **Cardiovascular disease risk**
- Blood pressure
- Body mass index
- Body composition (% body fat)
- Smoking habits
- Exercise habits
- Stress level
- Dietary fat intake
- Serum lipid profile
    (i) Total cholesterol
    (ii) High density lipoprotein
    (iii) Low density lipoprotein
- **Occupation-specific**
- Physical performance
    (i) Upper body muscle strength
    (ii) Abdominal muscle strength
    (iii) Aerobic fitness
    (iv) Flexibility
    (v) Job-related task performance time
- Pulmonary function
- Hearing acuity
- **Non-occupational medical-related costs and utilization**
- Inpatient
    (i) Number of inpatient admissions
    (ii) Average inpatient length of stay
    (iii) Cost of inpatient admissions
- Outpatient
    (i) Number of outpatient encounters
    (ii) Cost of outpatient encounters
- Productivity
    (i) Number of sick leave days used
    (ii) Cost of sick leave days used
- **Occupational medical-related costs and utilization**
- Number of occupational injuries
- Medical cost of occupational injuries
- Productivity
    (i) Number of days on leave
    (ii) Number of days on limited duty
    (iii) Cost of days on leave
    (iv) Cost of days on limited duty

for public safety and street and sanitation department workers, hepatitis B antigen and antibody status were checked in high-risk employees.

Cost-related outcomes of interest fall into two general categories – 'non-occupational related medical' and 'occupationally related medical', and encompass aspects of actual dollar amounts, lost productivity due to days off, and lost productivity due to limited duty. When evaluating cost-related outcomes, especially with regard to injuries, it is important to consider not only costs per employee, but also numbers of incidents per employee, occurrence rates for specific incident types, cost per incident, and cost per type of incident. Having this type of detailed information can help in interpreting changes observed in the distributions of certain outcome measures. As an example, we noticed an unexpected increase in the incidence of injuries in the most physically fit group of firefighters. Further analysis demonstrated that, while absolute incidence had risen in that group, cost per injury, amount of time lost per injury, average time lost per employee and average cost per employee remained lower than for less fit groups of firefighters.

Data collection in the field – incentives and practical approaches

After identifying the target outcome variables, strategies for collecting, managing and analysing the identified risks need to be put into place. One of the potential problems with collecting health-related data from a population is that people most interested in their health and least in need of reducing health risks are most likely to participate in health screening. In order to ensure the validity and, consequently, utility, of the occupational health information compiled, data collection methods need to incorporate strategies to guarantee that data are representative of the employee population. Incorporation of incentives for programme participation can help to lessen the bias that otherwise may produce distributions for the outcomes measured that do not truly reflect those in the employee population. Three types of incentives have been utilized within the City of Birmingham Good Health Programme to produce participation rates of around 95%:

- First, participation in the programme is made a requirement for taking part in city-sponsored and subsidized health insurance programmes, providing a strong financial incentive for participating.
- Second, screenings are made available on work time at a centrally located work site; accordingly, not only is the employee paid for the time involved in screening, but also no sick or vacation time is used up for the visit.
- Third, provision is made for employees who prefer to visit their own primary care health provider to obtain recommended health screening, with waiver of the insurance co-payment for the health-screen visit.
- Fourth, but by no means least, there is the use of a third party, not associated with the city, to administer the programme. This has provided a buffer between an employee's health information and his employer – guaranteeing that supervisors and other administrators do not have access to individual data, while meeting the needs of the

employer for programme evaluation of and justification for continued preventive service expenditures.

Within the Good Health Programme, data are collected in a variety of ways from several different sources. Two key elements of data collection that need to be considered are validity of the information and ease of entry. These elements are addressed by use of standardized training and certification protocols for data collectors (keeping human handling of the data to a minimum), reading original data files from a primary source directly into the health information dataset, evaluation of reliability statistics, and having extensive automated checking routines to identify unusual values. Specific examples of these approaches include:

- use of machine-read ScanTron mark-sense forms for direct entry of screening and fitness testing data, eliminating a separate keypunch step;
- directly reading medical claims data produced by the HMO accounting systems;
- directly merging injury data from the Occupational Safety and Health department database.

Data management and analysis – requirements and solutions

In order to be useful, the integrated database and analysis system needs to:

- handle a variety of data and data sources (e.g. text files, spreadsheets etc.);
- have the flexibility to add additional variables as required;
- track individuals over time;
- ensure data reliability and validity;
- facilitate data entry and maintenance;
- share data with various other programmes for specialized processing;
- incorporate safeguards to maintain individual confidentiality.

In order to meet these seven requirements, the Good Health Programme database and system was built around a core provided by the SAS analysis system (SAS Institute, 1996), which provides database management, data analysis and a common reference format for importing and exporting data of diverse configurations from and to other, more specialized programmes.

In terms of programme planning and evaluation, outcome measures need to be evaluated in relation to:

- change over time;
- changes compared with national and/or state trends;
- current values in relation to target goals.

If sufficient observations are available, inferential statistical tests can be utilized to see if there are significant changes over time, and/or to determine if observed changes are consistent with or better than reported national or state statistics. This last point is especially important in terms of evaluating programme effectiveness. Most programmes are instituted without use of an experimental design. Employees either self-select for participation, producing a non-equivalent control group, or everyone is exposed in the workplace to at least some part of the programme. Without a true control group, which would reflect changes occurring 'naturally' in the community as a whole, it may be misleading to ascribe observed changes in outcome measures to the effects of the occupational health and safety programme when, at best, only a portion of the observed change is a result of the interventions. For example, with efforts to control medical costs and the shift to HMOs for health care coverage, the rate of growth in medical expenditures per capita in the USA has been slowing. An occupational health and safety programme may realistically only take credit if employee per capita medical expenditures have increased more slowly than those for the USA in general.

Statistical methods can also be employed to set programme goals. Projection techniques can be used to extrapolate changes over, say, a five- or ten-year period. Because an employee population may have different characteristics than the population used to set national or state health goals, those goals may be inappropriately high or low for the employee population. Projections obtained using data collected from employees can be used to set realistic programme-outcome goals. Even in cases where inferential statistical methods are impractical, graphical presentations of data can provide a descriptive means for setting goals and evaluating progress toward these goals.

Concluding remarks

In conclusion, evaluation of a comprehensive occupational health and safety programme requires extensive commitment to the development and utilization of a database. Only through outcome evaluation, based on relevant measures, can OHS be evaluated, and directions for future improvements set.

References

Alabama Department of Public Health (1994) *1994 BRFSS Report.*

Brown, K., Hilyer, J., Artz, L., Glasscock, L. and Weaver, M. (1995) The Birmingham Good Health Program: Meeting *Healthy People 2000* objectives. *Health Values*, **19**(6), 45–53.

Forrester, B., Weaver, M., Brown, K., Phillips, J. and Hilyer, J. (1996) Personal health risk predictors of occupational injury among 3415 municipal employees. *J. Occup. Med.*, **38**(5), 515–21.

Health Care Financing Administration. (1996) *1996 HCFA statistics.* US Bureau of Data Management. Publication No. 03394.

Harvey, M., Whitmer, R., Hilyer, J. and Brown, K. (1993) The impact of a comprehensive medical benefit cost management programme for the city of Birmingham: Results at five years. *Am. J. Hlth Prom.*, **7**, 296–303.

Hilyer, J. and Artz, L. (1992) Physical fitness for emergency responders. In: *Emergency Responders Training Manual.* Center for Labor Education and Research. New York: Van Nostrand Reinhold.

Kizer, K, Pelletier, K. and Fielding, J. (1995) Work-site health promotion programmes and health care reform. *West. J. Med.*, **162**, 467–8.

SAS Institute, Inc. (1996). *The SAS System for Windows*. Cary, NC: SAS Institute.

US Department of Health and Human Services (1991) *Healthy People 2000: National Health Promotion and Disease Prevention Objectives*. Publication No. (PHS) 91-50212. Washington, DC: US GPO.

Weaver, M., Forrester, B., Brown, K., Phillips, J., Hilyer, J. and Capilouto, E. (1998) Health risk influence on medical care costs and utilization among 2, 898 employees. *Am. J. Prev. Med.* Oct, **15**(3), 250–253.

12

The new concept of 'Good OHS Practice' – the Finnish case

Kaj Husman and Matti Lamberg

The Finnish Ministry of Social Affairs and Health has – in conjunction with social partners to the labour market, providers of services and researchers – developed the Finnish occupational health services (OHS) system. A Governmental Ordinance has recently been issued which includes the new concept of 'Good Occupational Health Service Practice'. The concept covers local and national follow-up, evaluation and continuous quality improvement with regard to OHS.

Background

In 1990, a policy discussion was started within the Finnish Ministry of Social Affairs and Health on the adjustment of work to meet the needs and work ability of ageing workers. In 1991, a new paragraph was added to the Finnish Occupational Health Services Act (of 1978) concerning early rehabilitation. The concept of 'maintenance of work ability' was given legal status.

In the early 1990s, coverage of the paid workforce by the occupational health services (OHS) in Finland was 90% (according to annual surveys performed 1991–96). Although coverage was high, there was great variation in the quality of OHS offered by different providers and units. Changes in working life and the introduction of market economy ideas into the health care system in Finland raised a number of questions:

- What are the benefits of OHS for different types of enterprises and their workers?
- Does the OHS system meet the needs and demands of a changed working life?
- More specifically, do OHS units in the field satisfy the needs of their customers, workers and enterprises?

The National Advisory Board for OHS – a cooperative body representing labour market partners, providers of OHS, researchers at the Finnish Institute of Occupational Health (FIOH) and government authorities –

made a reform proposal with regard to OHS policy to the Ministry of Social Affairs and Health.

It was affirmed that activities stipulated by the 1978 Act on OHS had already been fairly well implemented. Nevertheless, there should be a new emphasis on development, focusing on the local needs of OHS customers and improvement of the quality of OHS practice. Accordingly, the Finnish Council of State introduced a new Governmental Ordinance on OHS. The new concept of 'Good Occupational Health Service Practice' (GOHSP) was introduced. Special emphasis was placed on the importance of activities for maintaining work ability. Further, a new model for the follow-up and evaluation of the Finnish OHS system was created.

The concept of Good Occupational Health Service Practice (GOHSP)

The Ordinance of the Council of State on OHS defines the aims of Good Occupational Health Service Practice (GOHSP) as providing for:

- a healthy and safe work environment;
- a well-functioning work organization;
- the prevention of work-related diseases;
- the maintenance and promotion of work ability;
- continuous quality improvement and evaluation of the effectiveness of OHS.

The inclusion of two of the 'new' objectives – 'a well-functioning work organization' and 'the maintenance and promotion of work ability' implies the need to expand the field of operation and range of skills of OHS providers. The third new task/concept – 'continuous, quality improvement and evaluation of the effectiveness of OHS' – emphasizes that responsibility to fulfil the requirements of GOHSP rests on all parties in working life. These include society (through legislation), employers (work-related factors), employees (work-related factors, behavioural aspects, life styles) and OHS (coordination, cooperation and expert services). Since they jointly formulated the concept on the National Advisory Board for OHS during the drafting of the Ordinance, all these parties have implicitly accepted GOHSP principles.

The Governmental Ordinance of the Council of State on OHS defines GOHSP methods as encompassing:

- workplace surveys;
- provision of information;
- counselling;
- health examinations;
- risk assessment;
- maintenance of first-aid skills;
- activities maintaining work ability;
- curative care (provisional).

Perhaps the most important aspect is that the concept of GOHSP entails that OHS must be:

- ethical, effective and of high quality;
- delivered by a multidisciplinary team;
- capable of undertaking carefully planned activities together with OHS customers, based on customers' needs and expectations;
- able to follow up and evaluate effects and quality of OHS processes;
- performed in close collaboration with workplaces (customer orientation).

The core principles of GOHSP

The activities of OHS, based on the GOHSP concept, had to be extended to all workplaces – irrespective of industry, and size or location of the enterprise. The Finnish health service has a tradition of strong central administration. Direction and control have been extremely detailed, and even regarded as an obstacle to the development of responses to the needs of changing society and working life.

Within public health care, this has led to a re-examination of the relative financing burdens of local municipalities and the state. In a reorganization of financing, efforts were made to move from the established state subsidy system – based on consumption of services – to fixed state subsidies, calculated according to population by municipality. At the same time, in 1993, central direction and control was lightened, and local decision-making and the development of health care activities on the basis of local needs and expectations were emphasized. Much normative central control has been replaced by information control.

In a similar way, the compensation system based on consumption of services was abandoned in relation to OHS. The centralized follow-up and compensation system, which extended to details and practical measures, was transformed into a support system encouraging the development of services in the workplace according to local needs. Public financing from the national sickness insurance system is now restricted to a certain maximum capitation-based reimbursement per employee.

The reform of reimbursement policy in OHS and related legal amendments (1994) provide good opportunities for improving the quality of OHS. But the implementation of a national policy for OHS requires reliable follow-up systems to be effective. These should be based on the development of 'own work' in the provision of services, which in turn demands acceptable methods for the follow-up of service quality (through audits and a national evaluation system).

To achieve the objectives of GOHSP requires close cooperation between workers and employers, so that the best possible ways of reaching occupational health goals can be found together. Good planning and follow-up of OHS activities are also needed. Not only outputs but also the outcomes, effectiveness and impacts of OHS must be continually evaluated by both providers and customers at local level.

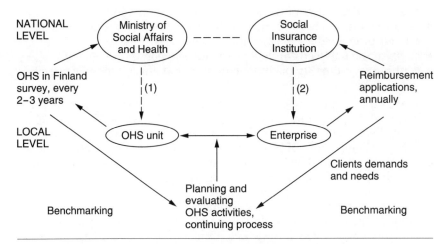

(1) Goal for the control and regulation: to ensure appropriate content, good occupational
    health practice, continuous quality improvement activities with outcome measurements
(2) Goal for the control and regulation: to ensure appropriate use of reimbursement funds

Figure 12.1 *The new follow-up system for OHS in Finland*

At national level, follow-up of OHS has been organized by the Ministry of Social Affairs and Health. A questionnaire survey covering the needs of enterprises and the inputs, process and outputs of all Finnish OHS units is performed every two or three years by the Research and Development Centre for OHS at the FIOH. National follow-up of the quality of OHS is also possible through scrutiny of the annual applications for reimbursement of OHS costs (50% of accepted cost) made by employers to Finland's National Social Security Institution. Figure 12.1 shows how continuous follow-up of Finnish OHS is now organized at local and national level.

It is of key importance that local level actions, including planning and evaluation, lead to better and more effective collaboration between clients (enterprise, workers, employers) and also to development of the activities of OHS. If this system were to be combined, as it should, with the ISO-based or some other quality system, it would lead to Continuous Quality Development (CQD).

Implementation and commitment

The new Governmental Ordinance of the Council of State on OHS came into force in 1995. At that time, there were no guidelines for, or any detailed descriptions of, the practical implementation of GOHSP. Nevertheless, the Ordinance clearly laid down the general principles to apply. In particular, these principles concern demands on providers of OHS. These involve:

• securing sufficiency of resources;

- goal-oriented nature of work and customer orientation;
- emphasizing central elements in the work process, professional status and requirements for the providers of services;
- cooperation between employers and employees;
- continuous follow-up of content, quality and effectiveness of activities.

Rather than providing detailed lists of measures for the legal provision of GOHSP, implementation was initiated in two ways. First, in 1995, a large development experiment was started in 50 OHS units together with the R&D Centre for OHS of the FIOH. The main objectives of the experiment were to develop quality management, activities maintaining work ability, OHS for small-scale enterprises, and follow-up of OHS activities, so that development activities were performed by OHS unit personnel together with their customers. Secondly, again in 1995, the writing of the GOHSP guideline manual was embarked upon. Seventy-two providers of OHS (physicians, nurses, physiotherapists, psychologists, occupational hygienists), FIOH experts and the Ministry of Social Affairs and Health were involved.

The GOHSP guidelines were published in the autumn of 1997, having gone through a consensus procedure involving the National Advisory Board for OHS. They were then distributed to all OHS units in Finland. In 1998, the FIOH started an extensive training project directed at all OHS units, with the aim of providing an in-depth introduction to the guidelines. OHS professionals and their customers' representatives are now actively participating in the training process. Simultaneously, a process to create detailed practice guidelines for different OHS activities has been initiated in conjunction with providers of the services, the FIOH and the Ministry.

Concluding remarks

The concept of 'Good Occupational Health Service Practice' has been introduced in Finland as part of a reform effected in close collaboration with all parties involved in occupational health and safety issues. It is not very common for the views of researchers and services providers to be taken into account in the formulation of an ordinance in this way. After the Ordinance came into force, a GOHSP guideline manual was prepared, and published in 1997. A frame of reference for good quality OHS has been determined at legislative level. It includes Continuous Quality Development of OHS in the field, and the evaluation and follow-up of services. An internal process to develop the functions and activities of OHS should now be carried out in workplaces and in OHS units – with the expert assistance, including training, of the FIOH. Good Occupational Health Service Practice can be implemented so that the points of views of customers (employees, employers, enterprises and authorities) are taken into account as well as quality, effectiveness, ethics, multi-disciplinarity and economics with regard to OHS.

Reference

Ministry of Social Affairs and Health, Finnish Institute of Occupational Health (1997) *Good Occupational Health Service Practice. Guidelines for planning and evaluation of activities.* (Hyvä työterveyshuoltokäytäntö. Opas toiminnan suunnitteluun ja seurantaan). Helsinki: FIOH (in Finnish).

13

Evaluation of OHS as a system of incentives – a German example

Johann Behrens

This chapter considers Donabedian's system model of evaluation of OHS in an economic perspective – in particular with regard to the impacts of supply-based and demand-based factors on health outcomes. An emphasis is placed on incentives for service production. Special attention is paid to possible theoretical and measurement deficiencies in relation to both process and outcome. The ideas involved are exemplified in research and surveillance settings, and then related to the concepts of evidence-based medical practice and quality.

Any evaluation of health care systems is – if sufficiently transparent and visible to its stakeholders – a system of incentives. Choosing wrong indicators of success or failure is likely to mislead responsible players, and may result in harm to clients. One reason for inaccurate indicators of effectiveness may lie in a defective theory or model for achieving desirable health effects. The system model of evaluation of OHS, according to Donabedian (1988), distinguishes between three aspects of health care quality – structure, process and outcome (see Chapter 2). These aspects are related to each other as links in a chain having an ultimate (and intended) impact on occupational health. In this view, the outcome is seen as a function of the process, and the process as a function of the structure. But it is essential to know the 'production function' in order to conceive what process will produce the outcome and the resources needed for an effective process.

Here, an economically influenced variant of the Donabedian model is proposed. The consequences of selecting inadequate output or outcome indicators are discussed, taking the example of evaluation of rehabilitation/'return-to work' programmes in Germany. Two further cases are commented upon – focusing on the relations between structure and process, and between process and outcome.

Hazards to evaluators of using wrong outcome indicators

As a basic principle, all health services should be managed in order to ensure high-quality performance leading to effective outcomes. In Germany, the trend in this context is to focus on the concept of 'Outcomes Management'. The current interest in evidence-based medicine (Raspe, 1998) and evidence-based nursing (Behrens, 1998) has contributed to a new emphasis on effectiveness and efficiency in all practice, and the need to have actions and practices grounded in research. Also, there is an increasing awareness that ineffective treatment or intervention may cause unnecessary harm to clients.

Figure 13.1 illustrates the distinction between process input and process output, and visualizes general programme outputs and outcome objectives.

Process inputs and process outputs are often only remotely related to intended final outcome objectives in terms of health effects. One of the

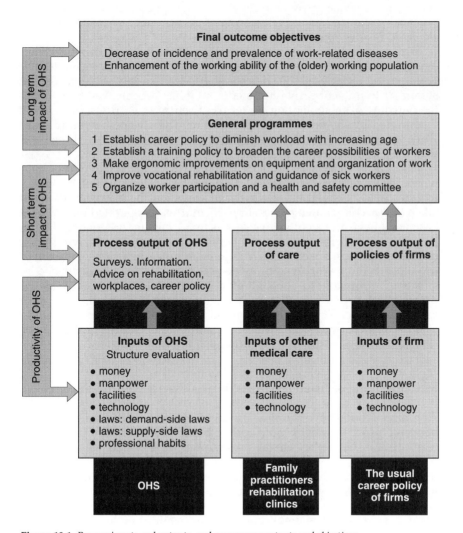

Figure 13.1 *Process inputs and outputs, and programme outputs and objectives*

main reasons for this is that, for effective action, the involvement of many players outside the health services is needed in preventive operations. Ultimate outcome objectives – such as decrease in incidence and prevalence of work-related diseases, health disorders and industrial accidents, return to work or enhancement of working capacity – are seldom achieved through action from Occupational Health Services (OHS) alone. An efficient and professionally operated personnel department in an enterprise may be expected to achieve such outcomes even with only a modest input from OHS. Figure 13.1 also shows the most important players and their resources.

Outcome objectives can be achieved without, or with very little, use of OHS. The health service units may function very well, all the right risk assessments may have been made, and consultations on preventive action and advice provided may be appropriate. Nevertheless, the practical actions taken in the enterprises do not seem to be effective and expected results do not materialize.

Further, selection of success indicators may be misleading. In Germany, the arena of occupational rehabilitation provides an example. The objective of rehabilitation, commonly funded by the social insurance system, is to prevent early retirement. But it has become well known that the outcome of rehabilitation (in terms of return to work) is, in practice, determined by the occupation of the client. The chances of returning to work are higher for white-collar workers, i.e. managers or civil servants, than for persons in blue-collar jobs.

This means that assessment of the success of a rehabilitation clinic, when using return to work as an outcome criterion, may be totally inaccurate if the selection of clients for treatment or intervention is not taken into account. Such clinics, in particular when operated on a market basis, will have an incentive to select as many clients for rehabilitation as possible from socio-economic segments in the population having good return-to-work prospects. They would be tempted to avoid admission of unskilled manual workers. Social inequality would than be deepened by selective admission to rehabilitation institutions – in breach of the principle of providing all persons with services, regardless of their income and social status (Behrens and Dreyer-Tümmel, 1994; Behrens, 1997). It is important to be aware of attempts to embellish health service statistics through restrictive institutional admission practices.

Measurement of inter-relations of process and inputs/outputs

As pointed out above, quality management should evaluate relations between process and output, and also pay constant attention to the relationships between general programme output and final outcome objectives. The time element is always important in such relationships. In all occupational health processes there may be both effects in a short-term perspective and long-term impacts on the health of clients. Here, it is important to be able to relate observations to an empirical model. If there is evidence of a long-term effect on health, quality management can focus on short-term effects and on input and output relations.

One example of a problematic outcome indicator is the sickness absence rate. A fall in reported sickness absenteeism may be brought about by many factors beyond the control of OHS and enterprise management. A reduction in the rate may, for example, be achieved by laying off employees with health defects (with a view to relieving the burden of sickness absence on the enterprise).

In view of the complexity – the wide range of differing endpoints and the multitude of factors bearing on the impact of preventive operations – any health evaluation is confronted by both conceptual and methodological difficulties.

Example: a study of compliance to national regulations

The German Work Safety Law is an example of public health regulation promulgated by the state but implemented by private companies with the support of health professionals (such as occupational health physicians). The two strategies commonly practised are:

- To invest on the supply-side, including provisions for occupational health physicians and their formal qualifications.
- To invest on the demand-side, including state regulations directly addressing safety-and-health management or corporate culture. Employers are commonly required to take action as responsible agents.

Behrens and Müller (1993) examined and assessed the workplace-related activities, as required by law, of a group of German occupational health physicians. Self-administered questionnaires were completed by 502 of the study population in 1990. This sample constituted one-third of a group ($n = 1500$) randomly selected from a list of 9602 physicians commissioned to carry out preventive health examinations. In addition, there were targeted interviews with 49 occupational health physicians, and participant observations for 15 days (with group discussions and feedback to members of the study populations).

Only one-third of questionnaire respondents reported that they in essence met the requirements of the German Work Safety Law with regard to workplace-related prevention. Since we wanted to know whether low compliance is due to supply-side or demand-side factors, a stepwise logistic regression analysis was performed. Independent variables included physician's formal qualification, years of experience in the profession, technical and staff provisions, gender and age.

Specific context or infrastructure of the OHS unit was regarded as a demand factor. Only variables indicating a prevention-oriented health and safety culture in a company – i.e. the presence of instructions on the handling of hazardous materials and permanent employment status of company physician – were found to be associated with a unit giving advice and recommendations on workplace-related prevention. The formal qualifications of the professionals had no bearing on the quantity or quality of advice given to the employer.

The study shows clearly that high qualifications are not enough on their own to enable occupational health physicians to comply properly with prevention-oriented, work-related legal requirements. More important are requirements on the demand side, such as state regulations that directly address the safety and health culture of the companies. Good qualifications of occupational health physicians should be combined with regulations and controls from agents external to the enterprise so as to provide a basis for an adequate preventive health and safety policy.

Example: the ASCA surveillance system

Over the past five years in the German state of Hesse, the authorities have developed a system (known as ASCA) for monitoring and auditing companies' safety and health protection systems. Objectives of the system are to analyse weaknesses in safety and health protection organization and to identify shortcomings in implementation of safety regulations. The system might help to evaluate the outputs and outcomes of the OHS units under surveillance.

A general checklist is provided for the employer. There are also special checklists for discretionary use – for external or internal health and safety experts and for OHS themselves. These may also be used by safety delegates, works councils and employees. The following questions are examined:

- Is there a basic understanding of safety and health protection for employees?
- Are people familiar with the duties and responsibilities involved?
- Are responsibilities clearly allocated and are they complied with in practice?
- Are there any systematic procedures?
- Are clear rules laid down, which work in practice?
- Are these rules comprehensive?
- Are the necessary skills available to the enterprise?
- Does the firm actively seek external advice and support?
- Is safety and health protection an integral part of company procedures?

Since 1994 the instrument has been applied in over 500 enterprises (50% of them having fewer than 200 employees, and 60 fewer than 50). The main results of surveys carried out in 1994 have been reported by Brückner (1997), and can be summarized as follows:

- Responsibility is clearly allocated and systematic checks carried out in just 9% of enterprises with fewer than 100 employees. In 30% of enterprises no checks are carried out.
- Employer's duties are clearly delegated and areas of responsibility defined in only 9% of small enterprises; 75% of enterprises have no such arrangement at all, while 19% of small enterprises have proper arrangements covering these aspects. In 49% of cases the application of official requirements was left to chance.
- Procedures for regular safety inspections involving safety experts in plant where surveillance is particularly necessary are laid down in only 9% of small enterprises; 67% have no such arrangements at all.

Relation to quality

Quality systems based on ISO 9000–9004 are mainly focused on compliance with internal structure and process standards. As part of its records, a quality system may provide information on client satisfaction. Any quality system of this type has until now not had its main focus on the impacts, effectiveness and efficiency of the occupational health process. One reason for this may lie in the implied assumption that the possible impacts of structure and process are already well known. Alternatively, it may be based on the notion that it is the client's responsibility to know what is to be expected from a health service organization. Both these presumptions are often not warranted. In fact they may be false. Even in the ASCA system there are only a few questions directly addressing or measuring the impacts of structure quality on process quality, of process output on general programme output, and of general programme output on achievement of final outcome objectives.

Concluding remarks

One of our problems as OHS professionals is that we consistently neglect the importance of having an evidence-based causal model of how a desired outcome is to be achieved. We are only too eager to focus on processes and process outputs. The varied interests of our clients contribute to this lack of specific focus. The fact remains that it is our professional duty to seek to identify the appropriate processes leading to final outcomes, and effective means with respect to health endpoints. Ability to achieve this would be a hallmark of professional OHS quality. Once an aetiologically targeted health service process has been identified, with reasonable certainty the next logical step might be to evaluate the compliance with standards of the kind available in ISO norms 9000–9004.

References

Albracht, G. and Brückner, B. (1997) Application of the ASCA system in small and medium-sized undertakings. paper for the SLIC Conference, Nordwijk.
Behrens, J. (1977) Krankheit/Armut. In: *Differenz und Integration* (S. Hradil, ed.). Frankfurt a.M: Campus, pp. 1054–74.
Behrens, J. (1998) Evidence based nursing in rehabilitation. *DRV-Schriften*, **10**, 394-5.
Behrens, J. and Dreyer-Tümmel, A. (1994) *Indikatoren der Rehabilitationsbedürftigkeit.* Frankfurt a/M: ISIS.
Behrens, J. and Müller, R. (1993) Supply and demand factors and compliance to German Work Safety Law. *Occup. Med.*, **43** (Suppl 1), 47–9.
Donabedian, A. (1988) The quality of care. How can it be assessed? *JAMA*, **260**, 1743–8.
Raspe, H. (1998) Evidence based medicine: anlässe, methoden, probleme. *Geburtsh und Frauenheilk*, **58**, M21-M25. Stuttgart, New York: Georg thieme Verlag.

14

Statistical implementation analysis of a public occupational health programme – the Canadian case

Diane Berthelette

The public occupational health programme of the Canadian Province of Quebec and the context of its implementation are described. The focus is on implementation analysis as a form of evaluation. A field study was conducted in order to identify the characteristics of the programme's process and client organizations associated with one of the programme's expected outcomes. The number of actions taken by firms exposed to the programme to reduce, at source, workers' exposure to occupational hazards is considered. Questionnaires were employed to gather data from the occupational health teams responsible for services delivery, and interviews to collect data from the firms exposed to the programme. Extensive statistical analysis of the data suggests that the programme is optimized locally through a combination of diversity of services on the part of local occupational health teams and cultural/structural characteristics favourable to primary prevention on the part of firms. A number of specific recommendations for improvement are made on the basis of results.

Essence of evaluation and nature of implementation analysis

The aim of evaluation is to produce knowledge that may be useful in making a value judgement about the whole or a portion of a programme – be it its objectives, its activities (process), its resources (structure), or its effects (outcome). Evaluation can refer to either a normative or a scientific process. Normative evaluation consists in the comparison of a programme's characteristics, selected in accordance with predefined criteria, with certain standards. For its part, evaluative research seeks to identify and understand the relations between programme components, such as the characteristics of services that produce the best expected outcomes (Contandriopoulos *et al.*, 1992). Accordingly, evaluative research contributes to the production of valid criteria and standards that may be used in normative evaluation.

The results of evaluation may be intended for persons in charge of the development, implementation and management of a programme – given that it is these individuals who will make decisions concerning its continuation, termination or modification. Research results may also be helpful to potential clients considering participation in future programmes (Contandriopoulos *et al.*, 1992).

The present chapter concerns the implementation, description and analysis of the public occupational health programme of the Province of Quebec in Canada. Implementation analysis can be regarded as a type of evaluative research. Whereas evaluation of a programme's results represents an attempt to verify whether it produces an expected outcome, implementation analysis attempts to identify the characteristics of a programme and the context in which it is implemented, both in relation to its results (Denis and Champagne, 1990). Formulation of the 'theory' underlying the programme and also an accurate description of its implementation are prerequisites of evaluation of this kind (Chen, 1990).

What we call the underlying theory corresponds to the characteristics of the process and structure of the programme. These are the characteristics chosen with a view to realizing programme objectives. In other words, they are the mechanisms that persons in charge of the programme use in order to produce expected outcomes (Bickman, 1987). However, since individuals who plan and implement programmes are not always aware of the theory they are applying, researchers rarely have access to documents that describe these mechanisms precisely and explicitly. This is why the researcher must often rely on an inductive approach – based on case studies – to arrive at a programme's underlying theory. Knowledge of this theory is useful in identifying the programme characteristics that should be included – as independent variables – in implementation analysis.

Further, researchers have noted that there can be a great difference between a programme as it is designed by its originators and the programme as it is implemented by those delivering the relevant services (Bickman, 1987; Chen, 1990). This difference may be at its greatest if there is considerable variability in implementing organizations, deliverers and clients (Scheirer, 1987; Chen, 1990). Accordingly, it is important to describe the operational characteristics of both implemented programmes and their client organizations.

These two stages – formulation of a theory underlying any programme and description of the implementation process – are prerequisites for the elaboration of an exhaustive theoretical model to be tested by empirical analysis. The model must also encompass external factors likely to have direct or indirect effects on programme results (Chen and Rossi, 1983). Reviewing the literature in the fields of evaluative research and organization theory may be a useful way of targeting these external factors.

The present chapter starts with a description of an occupational health programme that we have studied (the Occupational Health Programme (OHP) in Quebec), and the legal and social context in which it takes place. We then summarize scientific methods employed and evaluative results achieved in relation to the following objectives:

- to identify the criteria used by programme deliverers to define their intervention priorities;

- to describe variations in implementation, in other words to identify and compare the actual services provided by the programme (which is run by Local Occupational Health Teams (LOHTs) as mandated by the Quebec Occupational Health and Safety Act);
- to identify the characteristics of the OHP process and client organizations associated with one of the programme's expected outcomes – namely the number of measures implemented by business firms to eliminate occupational health and safety hazards at source.[1]

There then follows a discussion in which we compare and try to explain the similarities and differences that we have observed between the present and some previous studies designed either to evaluate the outcomes or analyse the implementation of the OHP in Quebec.

Finally, we comment on the scope and limits of our study, and make several recommendations for the improvement of both further studies and OHP implementation.

Study of the Occupational Health and Safety Programme in Quebec

The OHP under study has been in progress since 1981. It is mandated by the Quebec Occupational Health and Safety Act, whose stated purpose is to eliminate the root causes of work-related accidents and illnesses (Gouvernement du Québec, 1979). The key element in Quebec OHS policy is to place the responsibility for occupational health and safety on employers and workers. But small and medium-size businesses, which represent over 90% of firms in the primary and secondary industrial sectors (D'Amboise and Gasse, 1984), have few resources directly allotted to occupational health and safety (Pedersen and Sieber, 1989; Spiegel and Yassi, 1989; Berthelette and Planché, 1995). This is why the Quebec Commission of Occupational Health and Safety (COHS) – a government-related agency – entrusts Public Health Units (PHUs) with supervising the implementation of occupational health programmes in the enterprises operating within their respective regions (Gouvernement du Québec, 1978).

The basic components of the OHP are specified in Article 113 of the Occupational Health and Safety Act. In 1979, the COHS anticipated its gradual extension into various economic sectors, setting priorities on the basis of the frequency and seriousness of occupational injuries reported by firms in these sectors. By 1995, the year when we completed the acquisition of data for our study, the COHS had prioritized 15 out of the 32 economic sectors in Quebec.

In theory, only firms in priority sectors can benefit from the OHP

[1]This study was aided by two grants from the Fonds pour la formation de chercheurs et l'aide à la recherche, and the Social Science and Humanities Research Coucil of Canada, of which D. Berthelette is the Principal investigator. Ginette Lévesque (1997) did her masters degree thesis on the third objective of the present study. She received a masters degree grant from the Institut de recherche en santé et en sécurité du travail du Québec.

(Gouvernement du Québec, 1979). These firms are obliged to allow access to OHP deliverers; if they do not, the COHS can impose sanctions. OHP deliverers, however, only have advisory power; notices of dispensation and fines can only be issued by inspectors of the Commission. Accordingly, the relationship between OHP deliverers and their client organizations is prescribed and formalized.

The various PHUs created 15 regional occupational health teams to take responsibility for the planning, coordination and evaluation of the OHT. These regional teams delegate responsibility for implementation of local programmes to 73 Local Occupational Health teams (LOHTs) located in Local Community Service Centres.

The COHS has attempted to standardize the services provided by LOHTs. The Commission has defined – in the form of a contract – the nature of the services to be provided, the target clientele, and the magnitude of human and financial resources to be allotted to each team. It grants an average of 50 million Canadian dollars per year to OHP (Commission de la santé et de la sécurité du travail, 1998). These funds are used primarily to remunerate personnel in the multidisciplinary health teams, which include experts in the fields of occupational medicine and nursing, industrial hygiene and ergonomics.

The results of previous studies (Comité provincial en santé au travail, 1988; Berthelette and Pineault, 1992) have indicated that LOHTs provide the services mandated by the Act, namely:

- medical and environmental surveillance;
- evaluation of first-aid skills and making first-aid kits available in each firm;
- information and advice about primary and secondary prevention.

Despite this, a normative evaluation carried out by Price Waterhouse (1987) indicates that a portion of the resources allocated by the COHS to LOHTs is used for activities that are not specified under the Act.

In fact, the organizational cultures of the Commission and the teams are quite different. The COHS, which is under the authority of the Ministry of Labour, is responsible for the application of provincial legislation on occupational health and safety, including financial management of the Quebec workers' compensation fund. By contrast, LOHTs are part of small organizations – relatively autonomous – that are under the authority of the Ministry of Health and Social Affairs. The mandate of these latter organizations is to identify and fulfil the socio-sanitary needs of their local communities (White and Renaud, 1987).

The underlying theory of primary-prevention services provided by LOHTs to business firms is that environmental, biological and medical surveillance should serve to identify the occupational hazards to which workers are exposed, and evaluate the importance of health risks in the workplace. In theory, LOHTs must produce environmental and collective health reports in order to:

- inform employers, employees and members of Occupational Health and Safety Committees (OHSCs) of the occupational problems they have identified;

- help employers and members of OHSCs to define their intervention priorities.

In addition, advice provided by LOHTs should help employers to elaborate and implement the local OHPs mandated by the Occupational Health and Safety Act. The theoretical aim is to eliminate the root causes of work-related accidents and illnesses. However, a programme may also include the provision of individual protective equipment.

Objectives of the study

The objectives of the present study were: (a) to identify the criteria used by programme deliverers to define their intervention priorities, (b) to describe variations in OHP implementation, in other words identify and compare the actual services provided by LOHT to business firms with the services mandated by the Act on Occupational Health and Safety; and finally (c) to identify the characteristics of the OHP process and client organizations, associated with one of the programme's expected outcomes, which is the number of measures implemented by business firms to eliminate, at the source, occupational health and safety hazards.

Design of the implementation analysis and sources of information

The study addresses local OHPs implemented in the firms belonging to the 10 manufacturing sectors placed in a priority position by the COHS. The Quebec Research Institute of Occupational Health and Safety provided a list of these firms, grouped by geographical area and manufacturing sector. We used a stratified random sampling procedure to draw 904 firms from the list. Each of the firms was contacted in order to insure against selection bias.

Following drop-out, the number of firms in the final sample was 629, distributed across 43 LOHTs. Note that according to Canada's Respecting the Protection of Personal Information in the Private Sector Act, LOHTs need written authorization from business firms to disclose information on the services that they have provided.

We gathered data from the LOHTs between July and December 1995. The information collected concerned both number of occupational hazards, and the intensity of workers' exposure – as evaluated by each LOHT at the onset of programme implementation and during programme process. For this, we employed a structured self-administered questionnaire that had been pre-tested for content validity among two occupational health teams.

In addition, we made use of a telephone interview in which the person responsible for occupational health and safety in each firm with a health programme answered questions on the firm's structural and cultural characteristics, and actions taken between 1984 and 1994 to eliminate sources of occupational hazards.

A dependent variable was constructed by summing the number of actions belonging to the following categories:

- substitution of hazardous chemicals;
- replacement or modification of machines and tools to increase safety or to reduce noise exposure;
- installation of ventilation or aspirator systems.

We collected these data between February and June 1994, having pre-tested the interview form in 15 firms in order to validate its content. The results of a previous exploratory study served to define the content of both instruments.

Two variables concern the OHP process:

- intensity of services provided;
- frequency of services provided.

Intensity includes the number of LOHT services relevant to primary prevention provided to the firm, and the ratio of the number of hours devoted to the firm to its size. Frequency is the annual number of phone conversations, mailings, visits and group and individual meetings between the LOHT and its firms. We hypothesized that OHP process was positively associated with our dependent variable.

In addition, we considered the following characteristics of client organization as effect modifiers:

- the importance for the firm's management to invest in the primary prevention of occupational disabilities;
- the length of service of the occupational health and safety committee (OHSC);
- the number of equivalent full-time positions dedicated to occupational health and safety;
- the position held by the person in charge of OHS.

We hypothesized that the first three variables, and the fact of entrusting a middle executive or a foreman with OHS responsibility, would enhance the positive association between OHP process and hazard abatement.

Finally, we controlled for the potential confounding effects of the following firm characteristics:

- number of occupational hazards;
- intensity of workers' exposure;
- firm size;
- percentage of workers unionized.

Figure 14.1 depicts the model, showing the interconnection of modifying factors, independent and dependent variables and control variables.

Given the multivariate character of our theoretical model, we employed structural modelling as a research design. The dependent variable was transformed – according to $y' = \log 10(y + 1)$ – to meet the assumptions of multiple linear regression.

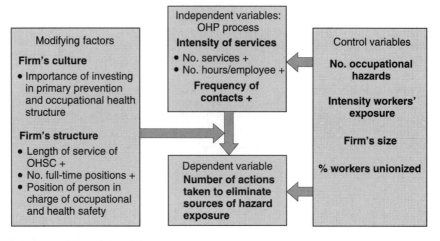

Figure 14.1 *Theoretical model*

Findings on OHP implementation

We obtained a 19.4% ($n = 122$) response rate from business enterprises. The response rates for LOHTs and programmes were 95.3% ($n = 41$) and 18.3% ($n = 115$), respectively. However, given the fact that some questionnaires were incomplete, the sample sizes used to describe and evaluate OHP implementation were 90 and 66, respectively.

Ninety-seven of 115 local OHPs had been introduced in the firms by 1995, indicating that the OHP implementation process had not yet been completed. Firms had benefited from LOHT services for 7.4 years on average ($s = 4.4$).

In most cases, the following criteria were considered very or extremely important by local teams in defining their intervention priorities:

- intensity of workers exposure to occupational hazards (98.8%);
- potential severity of health problems for workers exposed to an occupational risk (95.2%);
- number of workers exposed (69.5%);
- workers' concern about a risk factor (68.3%);
- the will of firms' management to reduce workers' exposure to occupational health hazards (57.4%).

Further, the priority attached to a risk factor or an occupational injury by the firm's OHSC was considered fairly to extremely important by 18.3% of the LOHTs.

Most of the local OHPs included evaluation of the number of first-aid workers and first-aid kits available in the firms (Table 14.1). According to Article 113 of the Occupational Health and Safety Act, one of the obligations of OHPs is to maintain adequate first-aid services. However, another regulation specifies that it is the employer's responsibility to provide first-aid kits and ensure that first-aid workers are properly trained.

We observed fairly high frequencies of activities aimed at informing workers and employers of the nature of risks in the firms, and also of preventive measures that should be implemented. The Act specifies that such services should be provided alongside medical supervision of workers. Biological surveillance is less frequent than medical surveillance. This result can be attributed either to low exposure to chemicals in the firms sampled or to the fact that few toxicological tests are available for early detection of harmful effects of chemicals.

The other services provided by LOHTs are not mentioned in Article 113 of the Occupational Health and Safety Act. Except for pre-employment examination, most of these services concern the main legal responsibilities placed on employers by the Act:

- implementation of the Workplace Hazardous Materials Information System;
- pregnant worker's re-assignment;
- protective re-assignment of workers who suffer from health problems;
- formation of health and safety committee;
- creation of occupational accident and illness prevention programme.

Finally, our results indicate that advice on professional rehabilitation and assignment of temporary work to persons suffering from occupational disabilities is provided by a small number of OHPs. The Act Respecting Industrial Accidents and Occupational Diseases specifies employer responsibilities on these issues.

Company size was always less than 200 employees, but varied considerably ($\bar{x} = 41.6$; $s = 47.5$). In addition, the mean percentage of unionized workers per firm was 32% ($\bar{x} = 44.9\%$), and the mean length of service of the OHSC was 3.7 years ($s = 5.2$). Less than 10% of the firms devoted a

Table 14.1 *Frequency of services provided within occupational health programmes (n = 90)*

Services	%
Evaluation of number of first-aid workers	100.0
Evaluation of first-aid kits	98.9
Advice on individual protective equipment	87.8
Advice on risk control	84.4
Environmental reporting	84.4
Information meetings with workers or employers	71.1
Medical surveillance	65.6
Collective health report	51.1
Advice on Workplace Hazardous Materials Information System	22.2
Advice on pregnant workers' re-assignment	21.1
Help to create Occupational Health and Safety Committee	17.1
Biological surveillance	16.7
Help to develop prevention programme	14.6
Advice on professional rehabilitation	12.2
Advice on assignment of temporary work	10.0
Advice on protective re-assignment.	10.0
Pre-employment examination	1.1

full-time position to OHS ($\bar{x} = 0.17$; $s = 0.38$); in 60% of cases, senior managers were entrusted with OHS responsibility (Table 14.2). Value attributed by firms' management to the importance of investing in primary prevention was 4.6 ($s = 0.9$). We measured this cultural characteristic using a Likert scale.

We employed a visual analogue scale in order to estimate number of occupational health and safety hazards, as well as intensity of workers' exposure (as evaluated by the LOHT at onset of programme implementation). The means of these variables were 4.6 ($s = 2.6$) and 5.1 ($s = 2.7$), respectively.

The mean number of primary-prevention services provided by LOHTs was 4 ($s = 2.2$) (Table 14.3). More than 75% of the firms received advice on actions to be taken in order to eliminate the root causes of occupational hazards, on environmental reports, and on the nature and importance of the risk factors identified by their LOHT. The mean number of hours per worker spent by LOHTs in firms since the start of OHP implementation was 6.3 ($s = 6.7$). The annual frequency of contact between LOHTs and firms was 8.5 ($s = 12.2$). Individual meetings with firm's employees was the type of contact most favoured by LOHTs.

An average of 13.5 ($s = 14.4$) hazard abatement actions were taken by the firms between 1984 and 1994. This result is markedly different from what we observed in 1989, when the mean number of hazard abatement actions was 2.4 (Berthelette and Pineault, 1992). Replacement or modification of machines to increase safety and installation of aspirator systems was the most frequent measure taken by the firms to reduce hazard exposure (Table 14.4).

Table 14.2 *Distribution of persons responsible for occupational health and safety by position (n = 66)*

Position	%
Senior manager	60
Middle manager	20
Foreman	6
Production worker	2
Clerical worker	12

Table 14.3 *Frequency of primary prevention services provided within occupational health programmes (n = 66)*

Services	%
Advice on risk control	81.8
Environmental report	78.7
Information meetings with workers or employers	65.2
Medical surveillance	59.1
Collective health report	43.9
Advice on Workplace Hazardous Materials Information System	24.2
Help to create occupational health and safety committee	19.7
Biological surveillance	13.6
Help to develop prevention programme	13.6

Table 14.4 *Actions taken by firms to eliminate the root causes of occupational hazards (n = 66)*

Type of action	Mean	s.d.
Replacement or modification of machines to increase safety	4.7	6.9
Installation of aspirator systems	3.3	7.1
Replacement or modification of tools to increase safety	1.3	2.9
Installation of ventilation systems	1.2	1.6
Replacement or modification of machines to reduce noise exposure	1.0	2.3
Replacement or modification of tools to reduce noise exposure	1.0	6.3
Substitution of hazardous chemicals	0.9	1.6

Interactions between one independent variable – the number of primary prevention services provided to the firm by its LOHT – and two modifying variables – the length of service of the firm's occupational health and safety committee, and the importance given by firm's management to primary-prevention investment – positively and significantly changed relationships with the dependent variable. The model explained 36.37% ($P = 0.00001$) of hazard-abatement variation.

We conducted a second analysis in order to test for main and interaction effects. We observed a positive statistically significant relationship between number of OHP services ($P = 0.0019$) and length of service of the firm's OHSC ($P = 0.0021$) and our dependent variable ($R^2 = 33.17$; $P = 0.00001$). Our results suggest that the value attributed to prevention by firm's management, and the length of service of its OHSC, influence the effect of OHP intensity on actions taken by the client organization to remove sources of hazard exposure.

Discussion

Our results indicate that most LOHTs adopt a public-health strategy to define their intervention priorities. They emphasize the intensity of workers' exposure, the potential severity of health problems that may result from hazard exposure, and the number of workers exposed. In addition, most LOHTs supply business firms with services mandated by the Occupational Health and Safety Act. Some LOHTs provide additional services in order to help their client organizations implement their own structures and programmes.

Advice on risk control has a higher frequency than environmental and medical surveillance. These results are different from those of previous studies in Quebec (Comité provincial de santé au travail, 1987; Berthelette and Pineault, 1992). This difference may be related to the experience acquired in the field of OHS by business firms – especially their OHSCs – since the earlier studies. Since OHSCs must contribute to the identification of hazards and means of primary prevention, firms may be more inclined to request advice on risk control. The synergy that we observed between number of OHP services and length of service of OHSC seems to support this hypothesis.

In addition, it seems that LOHTs now spend fewer hours per worker and initiate fewer annual contacts with their firms. The apparent decreases in hours spent and in contact frequency may be due to the increase in workload imposed on the teams since the COHS enlarged the size of their target groups. Without increasing LOHT size, five additional sectors were placed in a priority position.

The mean number of actions undertaken by firms to reduce sources of hazard exposure has increased from 2.4 to 13.5 since our first study (Berthelette and Pineault, 1992). But this difference must be interpreted with caution in the light of two factors. First, our original study was restricted to firms comprising a subsector of economic activity on the Island of Montreal. Second, between study occasions, we improved the construct validity of our preventive-action measures by including additional response categories in the questionnaire. However, it is also possible that the increase in OHP duration – in the firms belonging to the first five priority sectors – may explain the difference observed in the number of preventive actions performed by the firms.

The results of our analysis of the effects of the independent and modifying variables indicate that number of primary-prevention services provided is positively associated with number of hazard control actions. This finding is in line with an evaluative study of a public OHP designed for farmers in Finland (Vohlonen *et al.*, 1985). The Finnish researchers observed a positive, statistically significant association between exposure to OHP and farmers' knowledge of occupational health risks and improvement of their working conditions.

The present results, however, are different from what we observed in a previous study (Berthelette and Pineault, 1992). Length of service of the OHSC was the only variable significantly associated with number of hazard control actions. Differences in the study populations, in measurement of hazard-abatement actions, and in mean duration of OHP are likely to explain the discrepancies between the two Quebec studies. We can also speculate that modification of LOHT strategy is partly responsible for the observed difference over time in Quebec.

Finally, we observed that the importance attributed by business enterprises to the primary prevention of occupational disabilities, and the length of existence of their OHSCs increase the effect of the number of primary prevention services provided by LOHTs on the number of actions taken by firms to reduce the sources of workers' exposure to occupational risks. In other words, the expected outcomes of OHP are optimized when a LOHT diversifies its services in conjunction with its firms having cultural and structural characteristics that are favourable to primary prevention.

The results of the present study may be extrapolated to occupational health programmes implemented in business firms of less than 200 employees and which belong to the manufacturing sectors placed in a priority position by the Commission of Occupational Health and Safety.

The probabilistic character of our sampling procedure increases the external validity of our results. The response rate of occupational health teams is high (95%). However, the low response rate of firms (19%) may have reduced the statistical power of our analysis and jeopardized sample representativeness.

Spontaneous questions and comments made by firm managers who refused to take part in the study seem to indicate that most of them regard organizational factors in the field of occupational health and safety with suspicion. The need to sign a letter authorizing disclosure of information on services that their firm had been provided with seemed to increase suspicion. The concern was expressed that local occupational health teams and researchers may share their information with inspectors of the Commission of Occupational Health and Safety, in which case there would be a greater risk of being targeted by these inspectors. Finally, some respondents expressed their concern about the possible impact of the study. They feared that our results might jeopardize the autonomy of their team.

Concern about protection of anonymity and confidentiality of data and use of study results was expressed by many programme deliverers and their client organizations. Care was therefore taken to meet coordinators of LOHT to explain and discuss these aspects at the outset of study and to disseminate study results in study network. We recognize, however, the practical difficulties in communication on these matters directly with all client firms in a large study such as this.

Nevertheless, it is important to remember that evaluative research and organizational studies using probabilistic samples are scarce. In addition, structural models are rarely employed in organizational studies; case studies involving less than 20 firms and qualitative analysis are much more common.

Concluding remarks

Our results seem to indicate that the efficiency of occupational health programmes increases with the diversity of the services they provide, the importance client organizations attribute to the primary prevention of occupational disabilities and the length of existence of their occupational health and safety committee.

We recommend that local occupational health teams diversify the primary-prevention services they provide, and support firms in the implementation of their occupational health and safety committees. In addition, we suggest that the teams develop and implement occupational health-promotion programmes targeting firms' managers.

Further research is needed to estimate the impact that the implementation of these recommendations may have on the structure of health teams and the penetration rate of programmes in prioritized firms. The budget allowed by government-related agencies would probably need to be increased.

References

Berthelette, D. and Pineault, R. (1992) Analyse d'implantation du programme de santé au travail. Résultats d'une recherche évaluative. *Travail Santé*, **8** (4), S23–S30.

Berthelette, D. and Planché, F. (1995) *Évaluation de programmes de sécurité du travail dans des petites et moyennes entreprises*. Montréal: Institut de recherche en santé et en sécurité du travail.

Bickman, L. (1987) *Using Programme Theory in Evaluation. New Directions for Programme Evaluation*. San Francisco: Jossey–Bass.

Chen, H.-T. (1990) *Theory-driven Evaluations*. Newbury Park, CA: Sage Publications.

Chen, H.-T. and Rossi, P.H. (1983) Evaluating with sense. The theory-driven approach. *Eval. Rev.*, **7** (3), 283–302.

Comité provincial en santé au travail des Départements de santé communautaire de l'Association des Hôpitaux du Québec (1988) *Bilan des réalisations des services de santé. Opération Bilan 1987*. Montreal.

Commission de la santé et de la sécurité du travail (1998) *Rapport annuel 1997*. Montreal.

Contandriopoulos, A.-P., Champagne, F., Denis J.-L. and Pineault, R. (1992) *L'évaluation dans le domaine de la santé*. Montreal : Groupe de recherche interdisciplinaire en santé.

D'Amboise, G. and Gasse, Y. (1984) *La PME manufacturière 12 cas québécois*. Montreal: Gaétan Morin.

Denis, J.-L. and Champagne, F. (1990) L'analyse de l'implantation: modèles et méthodes. *Can. J. Progr. Eval.*, **5** (2), 47–67.

Gouvernement du Québec (1978) *Santé et sécurité du travail : politique québécoise de la santé et de la sécurité des travailleurs*. Quebec: Éditeur officiel du Québec.

Gouvernement du Québec (1979) *Loi sur la santé et la sécurité du travail, LRQ, Chapitre S2.1*. Quebec; Éditeur officiel du Québec.

Lévesque, G. (1997) *Les effets du programme québécois de santé au travail sur l'élimination des sources de danger*. Mémoire de maîtrise déposé au Programme de maîtrise en administration des affaires (profil recherche). Montreal: Université du Québec à Montréal.

Pedersen, D.H. and Sieber, W.K. (1989) Some trends in worker access to health care in the United States (1974–1983). *Am. J. Ind. Med.*, **15**, 151–65.

Price Waterhouse (1987) *Rapport final de la vérification intégrée du programme de santé au travail de la Commission de la santé et de la sécurité du travail du Québec*. Unpublished document. Montreal.

Scheirer, M.A. (1987) Programme theory and implementation theory: implications for evaluators. In: *Using Programme Theory in Evaluation* (L. Bickman, ed.). San Francisco: Jossey–Bass, pp. 59–76.

Spiegel, J. and Yassi, A. (1989) Community health centre based occupational health services for the small workplace: an Ontario study of employer acceptability. *Can. J. Publ. Hlth*, **80** (5), 355–8.

Vohlonen, I., Husman, K., Kalimo, E. *et al.* (1985) Occupational health services for farmers: A study based on an experiment in 1979–83. English summary. In: *Publications of the Social Insurance Institution*. Helsinki: Finland, A:21, pp. 199–217.

White, M. and Renaud, M. (1987) The involvement of the Public Health Network in Occupational Health and Safety: a strategic analysis. In *Commission d'enquête sur les services de santé et les services sociaux* (Gouvernement du Québec, ed.). Recherche 21.

15

Process evaluation of OHS rehabilitation work – a Swedish case

Ewa Menckel and Peter Westerholm

Different methods for data collection and a variety of feedback procedures were used to conduct a process-oriented evaluation of resources and activities with regard to the rehabilitation work of Occupational Health Services (OHS) in a Swedish enterprise. Interviews with OHS personnel and other interested parties, on-going registration of OHS contacts and activities, questionnaires to rehabilitated workers and their supervisors, and group discussions with OHS personnel were all employed. The study covered a variety of players in the rehabilitation process and highlights the importance of having both a summative and a formative evaluation approach.

OHS and rehabilitation in Sweden

Rehabilitation is a key task of occupational health services (OHS) in Sweden, with several government reports and committees, between 1990 and 1993, stating that the main focus of OHS work should be on prevention and rehabilitation. Changes to Sweden's Work Environment Act in July 1991 placed even greater emphasis on rehabilitation, and on OHS supporting employers with relatively new responsibilities in this arena.

This chapter examines OHS rehabilitation in Sweden by means of a process-oriented evaluation of the rehabilitation activities of a large in-house OHS unit at a major Swedish manufacturing company (Menckel *et al.*, 1996). The background to the study and the kind of evaluation chosen are briefly presented, followed by an account of the evaluation's aims, design, application and a selection of results. The main focus of the paper is on methods for data collection, where a process-oriented approach was adopted. Evaluation of OHS rehabilitation outcome was not included as part of the protocol.

OHS and the rehabilitation project

The OHS unit under consideration has responsibility for the work environment and health of workers in five workplaces, and is affiliated to one of Sweden's largest pulp and paper manufacturers, Svenska Cellulosa Aktiebolag (SCA), with headquarters 500 km north of Stockholm. Services provided are in the following areas: sickness absence and rehabilitation; health care and lifestyle; medical care and work environment. At the time of project implementation (January 1994), the OHS unit comprised three physicians, four nurses, one physical training consultant, one safety engineer and a chief administrative officer with accompanying staff.

The primary aim of the project was to promote rehabilitation capacity in SCA workplaces. The role of OHS was to coordinate various elements in the rehabilitation process, and to facilitate the return to work of employees on long-term sick leave. This involved collaborating with personnel in five workplaces and at four external rehabilitation institutions specializing in musculoskeletal disorders, asthma and respiratory diseases, alcohol and drug problems, and myocardial infarctions. Each institution provides care and training in its specialized area, for example: physical fitness programmes, advice on nutrition, adapted meal schemas, lifestyle programmes and self-development training and support are offered in the form of 2–6 week courses.

The concept of rehabilitation

A fundamental difficulty of rehabilitation and its evaluation lies in the wide variety of meanings of the concept of rehabilitation itself. Rehabilitation is usually regarded as encompassing a range of set measures that might restore the work capacity of individuals and enhance their opportunities for financial independence and self-support. This definition is extremely wide, and includes measures targeted at both individuals and the environment. The concept of working-life-oriented rehabilitation is used in this study to refer to **any actions taken in the workplace or by OHS that would promote the return to active work of an employee on sick leave**. The first priority in this context is therefore to **restore work capacity in relation to the current workplace**.

Players in the rehabilitation process

A variety of key players are involved in rehabilitation work, all of whom are likely to have their own focus which they regard as being especially important. They may be heavily involved in the process itself, e.g. a person receiving rehabilitation treatment, or participating in a more limited way, e.g. as primary care personnel. Figure 15.1 shows the various interest groups involved in ongoing rehabilitation work at SCA.

Whilst OHS personnel are the main focus group of this study, SCA employees undergoing rehabilitation, their job supervisors and personnel at the various rehabilitation institutions are also considered in the evaluation.

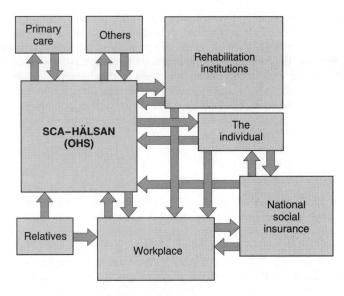

Figure 15.1 *Key players in OHS's rehabilitation process*

Selection of evaluation format

There are different evaluation formats, with a distinction often being made between contemporaneous (formative) and retrospective (summative) (see Figure 15.2 and further in Chapter 2; see also Weiss (1972) and Menckel (1993)). The process-oriented form of evaluation chosen for this study has both formative and summative features. The work process was monitored and documented as it developed (formative) and rehabilitation efforts were also discussed and assessed retrospectively relative to pre-set targets (summative).

A further formative aspect was that the information gathered during the project was compiled and fed back to the subjects of the evaluation

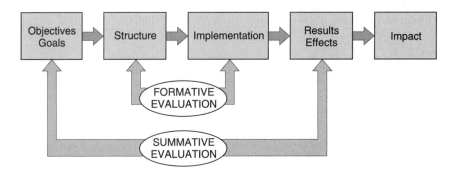

Figure 15.2 *Formative and summative evaluation in relation to the process of a project*

(OHS personnel at SCA) to enable them to discuss and amend their working practices. The formative evaluation also takes account of the influencing factors that result from the variety of stakeholders involved in the process. In this case, for example, the recipients of rehabilitation treatment along with their job supervisors and personnel at the various rehabilitation institutions were all covered by the evaluation. Their views on the work were collected and as this mostly took place after rehabilitation had been concluded, this information was deemed to be summative (see Table 15.1 below for further details).

The evaluation study: aim, scope and focus

The aim of this process-oriented evaluation study was to describe, monitor and analyse how a specific OHS unit in Sweden operated in the area of working-life-oriented rehabilitation in relation to five workplaces and four specialized external rehabilitation institutions. The evaluation was conducted by two researchers at Sweden's National Institute for Working Life in collaboration with OHS personnel. A nurse in the OHS unit liaised between the researchers and the OHS personnel.

The evaluation project focused initially on the rehabilitation efforts of the OHS unit at SCA (SCA Health) during the return-to-work phase of the process following attendance at a training course in one of the institutions. The project, however, was extended to encompass the so-called pre-admission phase, i.e. the phase during which SCA Health prepares for an employee's stay at a rehabilitation institution (e.g. through examination of complaints, contacting the institution or the workplace, and where necessary the next of kin).

The project was further expanded to include those cases of rehabilitation not sent to a specialized institution but treated by SCA Health itself, so-called 'regular' rehabilitation.

Evaluation methods and phases

The process-oriented evaluation focused specifically on OHS resources and activities (Rossi and Freeman, 1989), with different methods of data collection being employed during the various phases of the project (Table 15.1).

Table 15.1 *Data collection methodology*

Data collection methods	1993	1994	1995
1 Interviews with all personnel at SCA Health	Dec.		
2 On-going registration of OHS contacts and activities		Feb.—Dec.	
3 Interviews with personnel at the rehab institutions		Sep.	
4 Telephone interviews with OHS personnel		Oct.	
5 Questionnaire to workers			Mar.
6 Questionnaires to job supervisors			Apr.
7 Feedback to and discussions with OHS personnel		May	Sep. Nov.

Phase 1: Interviews with all personnel at SCA Health

Interviews were conducted with OHS personnel prior to implementation of the project to document how SCA Health had been working with rehabilitation in the year prior to commencement of the project. Expectations with regard to the project, and what a partly new approach to rehabilitation might entail was also evaluated: (a) for OHS personnel themselves (e.g. in terms of personal skills development); (b) for workers (e.g. in terms of return to work, enhanced life quality); and (c) for SCA Health organizationally (e.g. in terms of changed rehabilitation routines, increased contact with the workplaces).

Phase 2: On-going registration of OHS contacts and activities

Personnel at SCA Health were requested to fill in a specially developed form on every occasion they were involved in rehabilitation work. The two-page form (see Figure 15.3) contained questions about when and where contact was made, point in time and time devoted, type and principal nature of contact, and what measures/activities were agreed and decided upon.

Contact and activity form

Form filled in by:..

Date of contact: .... Time taken:.............

Information on the employee

Name:..

Born (yr mth day):...

Employed as:...

Workplace/company (even if outside SCA):.............

....

Rehab institution (if involved):...........................

....

A. Information on OHS's contact with:

employee	☐	other care-giver	☐
relative	☐	company	☐
rehab institution	☐	trade union	☐
primary care	☐	soc. ins. office	☐
specialist care	☐	other organization	☐

Contact person(s): name, position, and institution/ organization...

....

B. Form of contact

visit to OHS	☐	rehab group	☐
telephone conversation	☐	visit to workplace	☐
letter/fax	☐		
appointment/meeting	☐	other, please specify below	

....

C. Principal content of contact

treatment/therapy	☐
medical or social investigation	☐
individual-focused health care	☐
survey of workplace conditions	☐
family and other social conditions	☐
training/information	☐
personal finances	☐
other, please specify below	

....

D. Activities decided upon or agreed on occasion of contact

The employee contacts:

employer	☐
job supervisor	☐
rehab institution	☐
soc. ins. office	☐
other, please specify below	

....

....

Other activities/measures – to be taken by the employee

....

....

Other activities/measures – to be taken by OHS

Please specify by whom (which position)

....

....

Other activities/measures – to be taken by SCA

Please specify by whom (which position)

....

....

Activities/measures to be taken by other organizations/institutions

Please specify by which

....

....

E. New occasion of contact with the employee–OHS

within one week	☐
within one month	☐
on unspecified later date	☐
nothing agreed	☐

....

Figure 15.3 *OHS contacts and activities registration form*

Phases 3 and 4: Interviews with personnel at the rehabilitation institutions

Interviews were conducted with personnel at the rehabilitation institution specializing in back pain syndromes, and also during two study visits, the aim being to document contributions made to the rehabilitation process, especially contacts with SCA Health, and to record perceptions of rehabilitation work. Telephone interviews were also conducted with OHS personnel and the other rehabilitation institutions as the project progressed.

Phases 5 and 6: Questionnaires to workers and their job supervisors

At the end of the rehabilitation period questionnaires were sent to workers who had undergone rehabilitation and also to their supervisors. These contained items covering: contacts that had been made with SCA Health; which rehabilitation targets were regarded as most important; how measures decided upon were implemented and by whom; and the contribution of various players (including OHS personnel) to the process.

Phase 7: Feedback to and discussions with OHS personnel

One important aim of the evaluation was the feedback of information gathered to OHS personnel, so that they could discuss and change the ways in which they worked with rehabilitation (the formative part of the evaluation). The feedback took the form of group discussions between personnel and the two researchers, both during the project and after it was completed. The discussions were based in part on questions posed to personnel relating to information gathered in the phase 1 interviews and on information from the interviews with personnel at two of the rehabilitation institutions (phases 3 and 4).

The feedback procedure took into account the following crucial points listed by Whitman (1992), and applied by Menckel and colleagues (1997) in an evaluation study of the prevention of back injuries in Swedish health care:

- the importance of *credibility*, i.e. that feedback should only be provided when it is justified, and then preferably presented in a positive light;
- the importance of *responsiveness*, i.e. that all affected should have been given an opportunity to contribute what they know, and that there is a willingness to listen to the views of others;
- the key role of *trust*, i.e. that the receiver of feedback has sufficient confidence in the sender to understand and accept the message;
- the importance of providing feedback *at the right time*, i.e. usually as soon as possible after an event has occurred.

Accordingly, the feedback in this project concerning OHS rehabilitation work was only offered after all the OHS personnel involved had been given an opportunity to describe (in an interview or through the contact form) how they had acted. Providers of the feedback (the researchers) were 'trusted' persons, familiar with both the work and the project, thus ensuring: that feedback information was correct, that active participation was possible, and that feedback sessions were held with the appropriate degree of regularity.

Some data from the ongoing registration of OHS contacts (phase 2) and from the questionnaire administered to rehabilitated workers and their supervisors (phases 5 and 6) are presented below.

Results

The rehabilitation group

The rehabilitation treatment group comprised 117 workers, most of them men (approx. 80%), with an average age of 40–45 years (both women and men). Within the group 40% suffered from back complaints, 40% from asthma or other respiratory disorders and 5% from alcohol or drug problems; a further 15% had a multi-problem background diagnosis, including social and financial problems (later treated by OHS). Patients from the infarct clinic were not included.

Registration of contacts and activities

Over a period of 11 months, OHS personnel recorded 626 contacts with regard to 117 cases of rehabilitation, an average of 5.4 contacts per case. OHS physiotherapists formed the occupational group accounting for the largest number of contacts (40%), closely followed by OHS nurses (38%). Physicians accounted for 17% and administrative personnel 5%.

The maximum number of contact occasions recorded by any professional was nine. For one to three contacts, most forms were filled in by nurses; but for four or more, it was physiotherapists who recorded the most. For the first occasion of contact, around 30% of the forms were filled in by physicians, but this proportion steadily decreased as contact occasions increased. At the rehabilitation institution specializing in back syndromes, physiotherapists reported the greatest number of contacts, with nurses doing so at the other institutions.

OHS contacts were as follows: with the worker undergoing rehabilitation (57%); with the company/the workplaces (29%); and a smaller number with the rehabilitation institutions (5%). The average time taken for a single contact event was 20–30 minutes.

Contacts most often took the form of a visit to SCA Health (30%), particularly in cases of first contact (72 out of 117). Other frequent forms of contact included 'letter or fax', 'meeting', and 'special rehab group'. Visits to the workplace were made on 76 occasions for 117 workers, and were most often either the fourth or sixth contact made with the individual concerned.

The nature of contact varied over time, with the first occasion usually devoted to a medical/social examination, although the provision of training/information was also common. Training/information was most common on the second and third occasions, and surveying of the workplace was most commonly featured on the fourth.

On the first occasion of contact, the measure/action agreed upon was usually for the employee to contact his/her job supervisor or local social insurance office. This was suggested less often on the second occasion. It was also common on the first occasion of contact for a new meeting to be arranged within a period of one month. On the second occasion, new contacts were arranged for times as short as a week ahead, but no new appointment was generally made on the third occasion.

Questionnaire to workers and their supervisors

A questionnaire was sent to the 117 workers and their supervisors after rehabilitation had been completed. The response rate was 69% for workers and 66% for supervisors, with the rate of missing responses on individual items ranging between 0 and 5%.

With regard to perceptions of targets, 'coming back to the same job' was considered the most important target by both recipients of rehabilitation and their supervisors (48% and 51% respectively). The least popular alternative, for both rehabilitated workers and job supervisors, was 'coming back to the same work department'.

Among recipients of rehabilitation, 67% regarded SCA Health as having implemented measures agreed upon to a 'very considerable' or 'quite considerable' extent; 79% regarded themselves as having taken the actions that the measures entailed. The response pattern among supervisors was similar, although they stated without exception that all the measures decided-upon had in fact been carried out.

The rehabilitated persons and their job supervisors were also requested to assess the contribution of OHS to the rehabilitation process. Eighty per cent of recipients of treatment at the institution for back injuries stated that contact with SCA Health had contributed to a 'quite' or 'very' considerable extent to their rehabilitation. The proportion of positive responses was, however, lower among those who had received treatment for asthma or other respiratory complaints (50%), and also among those who had been treated solely at OHS without attending a specialized clinic (38%). Again, the assessments of supervisors were generally more favourable than those of workers.

Attitudes to whether rehabilitation had created better quality of life showed considerable variation between groups of rehabilitated workers. Those who had been suffering from disabling respiratory complaints were most positive, with 67% stating that rehabilitation had improved life quality. On the other hand, only 8% of those receiving rehabilitation solely within OHS shared this view.

Analyses and experiences

A variety of techniques for data collection and feedback were employed in the study to enable a process-oriented evaluation of resources and activities in OHS rehabilitation work to be conducted. The findings of the study are based mainly on: results from the survey of contacts made by OHS, the questionnaires administered to rehabilitated workers and their supervisors and group discussions with OHS personnel. Both summative and formative evaluation approaches were adopted taking into account the variety of players involved in the rehabilitation process.

By means of the survey of contacts (460 forms received) it was possible to examine OHS's extensive contact network, encompassing rehabilitated workers, workplaces and rehabilitation institutions. After a period of familiarization, these forms were regarded by OHS personnel as simple and not too time-consuming to fill in.

The information obtained from the forms was easy for the researchers to analyse, and then to feed back to personnel on various occasions. In this way, personnel were provided with a basis on which to discuss changes to routines and activities with regard to the rehabilitation process. One example is that, after a couple of months of registration, it became apparent that intensification of OHS contacts with workplaces had to take place, since these were not made by the rehabilitation institutions. During the feedback discussions, OHS personnel reported that greater contact with the workplace had facilitated return to work.

A general conclusion emerging from the project is that rehabilitation work is primarily the concern of OHS physicians, physiotherapists and nurses. Physiotherapists and nurses have a particularly large number of contacts whilst physicians seem to have the initial contact. Initial physician contact in relation to both workplaces and individual employees is generally followed up by nurses.

The results show that most of the workers and their supervisors consider that proposed rehabilitation measures had been considerably implemented. Most respondents also seem to regard the contribution made by OHS to the rehabilitation process as important.

It should be pointed out that the conclusions to be drawn from this survey have certain specific limitations. These are concerned with the skills profile and focus of interests of the specific OHS unit (SCA Health), the types of rehabilitation and the institutions involved, national (Swedish) circumstances, and so on. It should also be noted that this was a process evaluation by nature, designed to describe and follow the rehabilitation work of OHS rather than to assess the results of rehabilitation or the effects of actions taken (outcome evaluation).

Experiences from this study, and also subsequent analyses, demonstrate that it is important to adopt both a formative and summative approach to the evaluation of rehabilitation – the formative to exert influence during a period of change and to describe the contributions of the various parties involved, the summative to check whether various planned activities have actually been performed, and to assess results achieved. The importance of combining outcome (summative) evaluation with process (formative) measurement has been pointed to by Rossi and Freeman (1993) and Hulshof (1997).

The study confirms that effective working-life rehabilitation is dependent on the commitment of many different parties. The individual must be willing and active in seeking a path back to working life, but this must be accompanied by a resolve in the workplace to pursue meaningful rehabilitation activities. Perhaps one of the most important tasks of OHS is to ensure that such commitment is created. The process of evaluation is one of the key tools at its disposal in this regard.

References

Hulshof, C.T.I. (1997) Prevention and control of adverse effects of whole-body vibration - an evaluation study in occupational health services. Thesis, Coronel Institute for Occupational and Environmental Health, Academic Medical Centre, Division of Public Health, University of Amsterdam, The Netherlands.

Menckel, E. (1993) *Evaluating and Promoting Change in Occupational Health Services. Models and Applications.* Swedish Work Environment Fund.

Menckel, E., Westerholm, P. and Strömberg, A. (1996) *Arbetslivsinriktad rehabilitering – processorienterad utvärdering av en företagshälsovårds insatser.* Arbetslivsinstitutet, SCA–Hälsan, Sundsvall (in Swedish).

Menckel, E., Hagberg, M., Engkvist, E., Wigaeus Hjelm, E. and the PROSA study group (1997) The prevention of back injuries in Swedish health care – a comparison between two models for action-oriented feedback. *Appl. Erg.*, **28**, 1–7.

Rossi, P. and Freeman, H. (1993) *Evaluation: A Systematic Approach.* Newbury Park, CA: Sage Publications.

Weiss, C.H. (1972) *Evaluation Research. Methods for Assessing Program Effectivenes* (Methods of Social Science series). Englewood Cliffs, NJ: Prentice–Hall.

Whitman, N. (1992) 'Giving feedback'. In: *Effective Management of Occupational and Environmental Health and Safety Programmes* (R. Moser, ed.).Boston, MA: OEM Press, pp. 117–22.

16

Examples of occupational health audit – the UK case

Stuart Whitaker

This chapter describes the development of audit in occupational health in the UK, and identifies some of the driving forces that have shaped current practice. Examples of the audit of a vaccination programme and pre-employment assessment are used to illustrate the use of the most common model of audit. The advantages and limitations of such an approach are identified and discussed. In more broad terms, the status of standards used for audit and the basis used for setting those standards is highlighted as an important area for development in the future.

Background to the development of audit in the UK

Evaluation of clinical practice and audit has had a long history in the UK. The national survey of postoperative deaths is one example of a well-established evaluation of clinical practice. In recent years, however, there has been a dramatic increase in interest in audit and in audit activities across all health care disciplines. This upsurge of interest is principally due to a White Paper published by the UK government in 1989.

In the paper, called 'Working for Patients', the government states that:

> the government would like to see all hospital doctors taking part in what doctors themselves have come to call 'medical audit' – a systematic, critical analysis of the quality of medical care, including the procedures used for diagnosis and treatment, the use of resources, and the resulting outcome for the patient (Department of Health, 1989).

The government made substantial funding available to the National Health Service to support the development of medical, and later clinical audit, including funding for training programmes, individual projects and for administrative support. However, different specialties and professional groups were left to themselves to develop the most appropriate strategies and methodologies for audit within their own disciplines.

Some methods have worked better than others in practice, and most have been improved with experience.

The Royal College of Physicians, of which the Faculty of Occupational Medicine is a part, published its first report on Medical Audit in 1989 (Royal College of Physicians, 1989). This report emphasized the need for medical audit to be carried out by all medical practitioners, and for it to become accepted as an integral part of normal medical practice. Their second report (Royal College of Physicians, 1993) emphasized that the nature of medical audit was primarily educational, aimed at improving practice and not the detection of 'bad apples'. Although improving the use of resources for health care was considered to be an important part of audit and one of the benefits often cited, the control of costs was not seen to be the primary aim of medical or clinical audit.

It was quickly recognized by the Royal Colleges that the quality of medical care is not determined solely by doctors, but also by the work of other professional colleagues, such as nurses. With the support of the Royal College of Nursing the scope of audit was widened to include other health-care professionals – under the term of 'clinical audit'. Quality assurance and evaluation of practice was not new to nursing. The Royal College of Nursing 'Standards of Care' project has been in operation since the mid-1960s and has developed several useful approaches to standard-setting, quality assurance and methods for evaluating nursing practice (Royal College of Nursing, 1989). However, increased government attention to the quality of health care helped to promote audit and evaluation across all health care disciplines.

During the early 1990s, several key papers were published by occupational health professionals encouraging the use of audit in occupational health practice (Agius, 1991; Macdonald, 1992; Whitaker, 1994). In March 1995 the Faculty of Occupational Medicine published its first report on audit 'Quality and Audit in Occupational Health' (Faculty of Occupational Medicine, 1995). The title of this document reflects the direction in which audit, alongside the development of quality management systems, has taken in the UK. Unlike hospital medicine, occupational health has always been closely associated with industry, and therefore the efforts directed at improving the quality of occupational health services (OHS) have been closely linked to the strategies already being used by industry to improve the quality of their own services and products. Some occupational health departments have adopted the ISO-9000/BS5750 approach and have incorporated elements of both medical and clinical audit into quality systems. Others have been reluctant to seek ISO recognition, sometimes questioning the cost, relevance and value of the ISO approach, but it is fair to say that all occupational health departments in the UK have been influenced – to varying degrees – by the principles of quality improvement.

The common model for audit in the UK

The most common approach to clinical audit used in occupational health in the UK is based on Donabedian's 'structure, process and outcome'

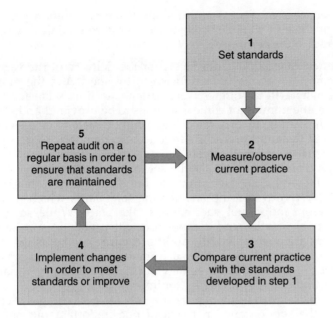

Figure 16.1 *The common model for audit in the UK*

model (Donabedian, 1966), which uses techniques such as the 'audit spiral' (Whitaker and Gardiner, 1995) to help set standards, observe practice and compare current practice against the identified standard. In this model, changes can be introduced to ensure that the consistency of practice is maintained or to further improve the quality of practice. The standards set should be subjected to a rigorous process of continuous review, which takes account of new research and information generated from the audit process.

This theoretical model (depicted in Figure 16.1) is based on a process of continuous quality improvement and as such can be incorporated, in theory, into a process of total quality management. In practice, there are a number of limitations to this approach (which are discussed at the end of this chapter).

Examples from current practice

The audit cycle can be broken into at any stage. For example, an audit programme might be developed at the same time as changes to clinical practice are introduced.

Example 1 – a vaccination programme

The introduction of a new hepatitis-B vaccination programme for health care workers will require occupational health professionals to consider the efficiency, effectiveness and quality of the vaccination programme. The vaccine itself will have been subject to rigorous clinical trials which are separate to the audit process.

- **Efficiency:** Standards could be set for the delivery of the vaccination programme, in terms of its efficiency, by specifying the number of people who will be offered vaccination, the time scale for the programme, the number of clinical sessions to be provided and staff to be used. This can be incorporated into a fully costed service level agreement, and the audit procedure used to help monitor progress towards specific pre-determined targets.
- **Quality:** Standards could also be set to ensure the quality of care, in terms of the clinical procedures to be used, the documentation required for record-keeping and for the safeguards which must be in place before individual vaccinations take place. While standards of professional practice and competence will usually ensure that these standards are maintained, the audit procedure can be used to demonstrate to clients and others that such standards are applied consistently in practice. Audit procedures may also help to identify variations in practice and offer opportunities for improvement.
- **Effectiveness:** Standards may also be set for evaluating the effectiveness of the programme, in terms of one important outcome – the number of people in a potentially exposed population who have been successfully vaccinated. A reduction in risk, for a potentially exposed population, is a legitimate outcome which can be used to measure the effectiveness of a preventive strategy.

The ultimate validator of the intervention, a reduction in the number of cases of disease, would be the most rewarding long-term outcome. However, this type of health outcome can be difficult to measure, and may be better suited to a well-designed rigorous research project, rather than through systems of quality assurance.

Example 2 – pre-employment assessment

An alternative approach is to start the audit process by observing current practice. This might be particularly useful where there is no good research-based evidence available on which to base standards. This approach was used in the UK in a national audit of pre-employment assessments (Whitaker and Aw, 1995). All occupational health departments in the UK National Health Service (NHS) perform some type of pre-employment assessment, but little information was available on the methods used to perform the assessment or on the outcome of assessments, in terms of the recommendations on fitness to work made by occupational health professionals following assessment.

The audit was designed to gather information on current practice and contrast the outcome of assessments performed by different methods. Information was gathered on the reasons for restriction and rejection. The questionnaires used to gather information at pre-employment assessment were subject to a peer-review process as a separate exercise (Whitaker, 1997).

The audit was performed by a randomized sample of 40 (18%) occupational health departments in the NHS, each of which provided information on a standardized questionnaire on all pre-employment assessment undertaken over a 3-month period. This produced 9139 questionnaire returns. Analysis of these data demonstrated that 98% of all applicants were considered 'fit for work': 120 (1.3%) individuals were assessed as 'fit for work, but with some restriction', and 65 (0.7%) individuals were considered 'unfit'.

The most common reasons for rejection were an abnormal body mass index (40%), skin conditions (21.5%) and psychiatric conditions (10.8%). The most common reasons for restriction were musculoskeletal conditions (27.5%) and skin conditions (15%).

The most common method of assessment was by a self-administered questionnaire alone (49%). A self-administered questionnaire followed by a nurse interview as standard practice was the next most common (34%). Referral to a physician was relatively uncommon. Comparing rejection rates by different methods of assessment showed that there was no significant difference between the use of a self-completed questionnaire on its own or when this is combined with a nurse interview as standard practice. Both methods of assessment allow for referral to an occupational physician where potential problems are identified. However, the use of an occupational health nurse to perform pre-employment assessments on all job applicants represents a significant use of this valuable resource.

A common approach to pre-employment assessment in the NHS – based on the use of a standardized pre-employment questionnaire, decision-analysis model and the introduction of an appeal process – was recommended in the light of earlier experiences (Whitaker, 1997). This audit provided new information on current practices and helped to focus attention on this particular occupational health practice. The discussions which followed publication of the results went beyond the scope of the study as more fundamental questions were asked about the efficiency, effectiveness, legitimacy and cost benefit of pre-employment assessments. The audit has led to changes in practice and has been used by others to focus attention on local issues.

Limitations of this approach to audit

In Example 1, the audit procedure began by setting standards for the efficiency, effectiveness and quality of a vaccination programme. However, there are a number of issues raised by this approach. Standards can be set at different levels – gold, silver or bronze representing the ideal or highest achievable standard or lower levels. In setting standards it should be made clear what the standard is intended to represent. If the standard is intended to represent an ideal, which practitioners should aspire to achieve, failure to achieve the standard may not represent a significant problem. However, failure to meet a minimum standard may indicate a significant problem. It is important that the standards that are set are understood by those who will use them, and an important step in designing an audit programme is to make explicit what the standard is intended to represent. It may also be useful to specify, prior to the audit, what action would be triggered by a failure to meet the standard.

Where targets are set for the delivery of a service and the performance of OHS is to be judged against specific objectives, it is important that these objectives can be achieved by the efforts of the OHS unit in question. In the example of the vaccination programme, the participation rate by employees in the programme may not be under the direct influence of the OHS. Accordingly, the performance of the OHS should not be judged by the participation rate alone.

Where standards are set for the quality of a programme, the measures chosen may reflect what professionals think are important criteria – clinical procedures, records, safeguards etc. But these may not be good indicators of quality from the perspective of employees. Other indicators – such as the explanation of the programme or procedures, reception at the OHS or availability of advice on other issues at the time of vaccination – may be more important to the employees. The selection of quality indicators should take account of all the stakeholders' interests.

In Example 2, the audit procedure began by observing the current practice of pre-employment assessments. While defining what current practice consists of is an important step in the audit cycle, in itself, this step may not identify good practice. Where there is no good research-based evidence available on which to base standards these are often defined as much by custom and practice, consensus agreement or perceived wisdom – all of which are open to debate. The crucial point when dealing with standards based on some form of consensus agreement is that there must be a very clear objective to the process that is recognized and accepted by all involved in the audit, otherwise the audit or evaluation of the process can become a meaningless exercise. Regardless of whether there is a scientific basis for the activity or not, unless there is a clearly defined purpose or objective set, evaluation of the activity against its stated purpose becomes impossible.

In conclusion, the audit procedure described here is the most common approach used for clinical audit in occupational health departments in the UK. While clinical audit can be used as a powerful tool to focus the professional's attention on what they are doing and can help to identify areas for improvement, each stage of the audit process can raise complex issues. Where a strong research basis for setting standards does not exist, an inherent weakness of the process is that practice is directed towards and measured against activities which have little or no evidence base to support them. Where standards for a particular activity have been set it can be difficult for individuals to challenge them. There is a danger that rigid standards might stifle new developments, unless those involved are prepared constantly to review their practices against new research findings and remain open to change.

The process of managing change can be time-consuming and difficult. Where there is little appreciation among the professionals involved of the need to change, or willingness to abandon traditional practices in favour of new or more efficient methods this stage of the audit process can fail. Ensuring that there is an awareness of the need for change, fostering a willingness to consider new approaches and maintaining the motivation of staff are important factors to consider when planning an audit. Otherwise, valuable time and resources may be wasted.

Another factor to consider is that where audit findings identify gaps in knowledge it is important to distinguish between quality assurance techniques, of which audit is one, and research. Quality assurance – those techniques which compare the actual product or service delivered against an agreed standard – helps to ensure that a consistent approach is adopted, and over time can help to improve the delivery of services. Where new questions need to be answered, a well constructed and performed research project is required. The two activities should not be confused.

There are many potential overlaps between research and audit. Research can be used as the basis for setting standards against which practice can be audited. Audit can identify gaps in knowledge – for example, about the effectiveness of certain practices such as pre-employment assessment – but research is required to investigate the effectiveness of those activities. Audit might utilize research techniques in observing current practices, by developing sampling strategies to ensure representativeness, statistical analysis of audit data, objective measurement etc. Research can be performed to evaluate the effectiveness of audit, and finally the data generated through repeated audits can provide the data for research to be performed.

The difference between the two is principally in approach and in the skills required to perform each activity. Where a professional or group of professionals possesses the skills to undertake both research and audit, there is great potential for high quality health services research and evaluation to be performed.

References

Agius, R.M. (1991) Peer review audit in occupational medicine. *J. Soc. Occup. Med.*, **40**, 87–88.

Department of Health (1989) *Working for Patients*. Medical Audit. London: HMSO.

Donabedian, A. (1966) Evaluating the quality of medical care. *Millbank Mem. Fund Q.*, **44**, 166–206.

Faculty of Occupational Medicine (1995) *Quality and Audit in Occupational Health*. London: Faculty of Occupational Medicine, Royal College of Physicians.

Macdonald, E.B. (1992) Audit and quality in occupational health. *Occup. Med.*, **42**, 7–11.

Royal College of Nursing (1989) *A Framework for Quality*. London: Scutari Press.

Royal College of Physicians of London. (1989) *Medical Audit. A First Report: What, Why and How?* London: Royal College of Physicians.

Royal College of Physicians of London (1993) *Medical Audit. A Second Report*. London: Royal College of Physicians.

Whitaker, S. (1994) Pre-employment assessment: working towards standards of good practice in the NHS. *Occup Hlth*, **45**, 412–13.

Whitaker, S. (1997) A critical evaluation of pre-employment assessment in the National Health Service. PhD thesis, University of Birmingham, Birmingham, UK.

Whitaker, S. and Aw, T.C. (1995) Audit of pre-employment assessments by occupational health departments in the National Health Service. *Occup. Med.*, **45,** 75–80.

Whitaker, S. and Gardiner, K. (1995) Audit in occupational hygiene. In: *Occupational Hygiene*, 2nd edn (K. Gardiner and J.M. Harrington, eds). Oxford: Blackwell Scientific, pp. 417–28.

17

Problem-based rehabilitation of work-related musculoskeletal disorders – a Swedish case

Kerstin Ekberg

A problem-based learning method for rehabilitation of work-related disorders and human resource development at work is described. By using such a method, the advantages of a high degree of individual control and influence, individually adjusted demands, and extensive social support can be utilized. Three levels of action in the rehabilitation process are approached – the work situation, the mediating psychosocial resources of the individual, and health outcome (including physical, social and psychological functions). Improved psychosocial resources – such as self-esteem, coping resources, and improved work conditions – are considered relevant to good prognosis following rehabilitation.

Perspectives on rehabilitation

Musculoskeletal disorders, in particular those affecting the back, neck and shoulders, cause the largest consumption of health care resources in the Western world. The difficulties involved in diagnosing musculo-skeletal disorders contribute to problems of understanding and exploring causes of the symptoms and how they should be treated.

OHS clinicians and physicians are faced with a number of different treatment methods. The method used most likely reflects the opinion of the researcher or clinician on causes of the disorder, and possibly also on the goals established for the rehabilitation process.

A medical perspective on the aetiology of any disorder may lead to treatment methods that are primarily aimed at restoring mobility and strength, and at reducing pain. A multi-causal perspective may prompt a wider range of treatment methods; the goals of the rehabilitation process will be more far-reaching, involving measures such as work ability, psychic well-being and social activities.

All this, of course, has implications for studies of the outcome of rehabilitation, since different perspectives produce different aims and treatment methods. A successful rehabilitation – on one perspective – may be regarded as less successful from another. Evaluation of any rehabilitation outcome must be determined by the goals of the rehabilitation process.

Prevention and rehabilitation appear to be more successful if not only external factors, but also internal, mediating factors – such as perception of work conditions, perception of health, and appropriate coping resources – are treated as important parts of the rehabilitation process.

The importance of acknowledging a patient's/worker's disorder (rather than neglecting it) must be stressed. Scepticism on the part of others may force patients into a pattern of credibility-seeking, which might maintain and prolong their illness. Sickness absence, for example, has been interpreted as a coping behaviour directed against strenuous work conditions and perceived ill-health. On this line of reasoning, work and psychosocial conditions that allow for efficient coping strategies in the workplace when demands are perceived as too high are crucial to a favourable health outcome. Social support and recognition by supervisors has been observed in several studies as important for primary prevention and for facilitating subsequent re-entry.

The negative outcome of many rehabilitation programmes may partly be due to the lack of control of compliance of the activities involved in the programme. Lack of adherence or compliance, which is a particularly common problem in rehabilitation programmes of longer duration, is often regarded as involving a lack of motivation on the part of the patient or employee. It may, however, be more fruitful to identify typical circumstances that are barriers to programme compliance.

Some common barriers have been discussed by McIntosh and colleagues (1995). They point to the importance of not only focusing rehabilitation activities on pain itself, but also on a rehabilitation programme being realistic and regarded as valuable by the patient. Return to unchanged work may be a less desirable goal for a patient who strongly dislikes the job, or who is involved in conflicts at work.

A general problem in most rehabilitation and intervention programmes appears to be the absence of a participative approach to establishing the individual's specific goals for rehabilitation, and also strategies for reaching these goals. In organizational psychology, participative models have been demonstrated to improve worker motivation and productivity. In the 'demand–control–social support' model described by Karasek and Theorell (1990), important aspects of work organization that promote health and prevent stress-related disorders are outlined. The model has gained extensive support in epidemiological studies of work-related stress disorders. Of particular importance for a favourable health outcome is high decision latitude at work, in combination with demands that do not exceed the individual's resources, plus good social support.

The combination of high demands and low decision latitude is a promoter of strain. It is suggested that a work situation inducing high strain may inhibit learning as a result of accumulated anxiety. By contrast, high decision latitude in combination with demands that are perceived as possible to cope with may stimulate ability and willingness to accept challenges and new learning.

New learning leads to a reduction of perceived stress and to improved coping, and – eventually – a feeling of mastery may develop as a global behavioural orientation. Similarly, worker participation and a high degree of involvement and support from management may promote a successful rehabilitation process by increasing ability to accept challenges and new learning. But, if the rehabilitation process and the goals for the process are pre-determined by experts, mechanisms enforcing passivity and alienation may be activated (Ben-Zira, 1986), and the rehabilitation process may yield a patient who is more passive and dependent than when rehabilitation started.

A problem-based model

In problem-based rehabilitation it is assumed that the worker is the best expert on how the rehabilitation process should proceed, and which goals for rehabilitation should be given priority in the short and long run. It is considered essential that workers themselves formulate the goals for their rehabilitation and develop individual strategies to reach these goals. By using a problem-based method, the advantages of a high degree of individual control and influence, of individually adjusted demands and of extensive social support can be utilized.

A heuristic model of essential components of the rehabilitation process is outlined in Figure 17.1.

In essence, the model points to three levels of action relevant to the rehabilitation of work-related disorders:

- the mediating psychosocial resources of the individual;
- the work situation;
- the health outcome (including physical, social and psychological functions).

From this perspective, aspects of the work situation and of mediating psychosocial resources are considered as equally important to a success-

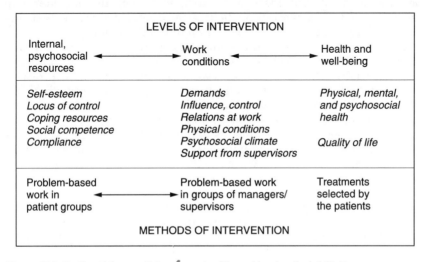

Figure 17.1 *Outline of the essential components of the problem-based rehabilitation process*

ful rehabilitation process as reduction of pain, increased muscular strength, and other physical outcome measures.

The problem-based method and its implementation

The method of problem-based rehabilitation is founded in problem-based learning (see Barrows, 1985), but adapted to the context in question. On this technique, employees with musculoskeletal problems work in groups for about two hours every week for about four months. There is a specially trained tutor in each group, often a professional from OHS, whose main task is to ensure that the group process is constructive. The tutor should not, however, get involved in the work content of the group.

At each meeting, group work follows the problem-based method. First, the group decides on a theme to discuss during the meeting – a theme which might focus on the work situation, on the situation outside work, or on internal problems. Examples of such themes are stress at work, hindrance factors, self-esteem, health, exercise and so on. The group then has a brainstorming session on the selected theme. If, for example, the selected theme is 'Work', the outcome of the brainstorming session may look as in Figure 17.2. The two examples displayed in the figure show differences in associations between a group with short-term periods of sick leave only (Figure17.2a) and a group on long-term sick leave (Figure 17.2b).

The brainstorming session in the group on long-term sick leave largely focuses on a bad psychosocial climate and relations with superiors and workmates. This gives a hint concerning the importance of hindrance factors for returning to work in this group.

The outcome of the brainstorming process is structured into content categories. During this process, the discussions between group members give rise to many new ideas and associations. Both the brainstorming process and the categorization help group members to see that any problem may be seen from several different points of view.

In the first case, the resulting content categories of the brainstorming session may be 'supervisory behaviour', 'physical work conditions', 'psychosocial work conditions' and 'work-related health'. By contrast, in the second case, the content categories may be 'relations with work-mates', 'relations with supervisors' and 'health'. The outcomes of the brainstorming and categorization sessions vary by group.

Having categorized the outcome of its brainstorming session, the group decides on one of the categories to proceed with, and each group member decides on an individual goal – related to the category – to accomplish prior to the next group session. If the selected category is 'supervisory behaviour', such an individual goal might be 'to initiate discussions with supervisor about lack of feedback'. It is important that these goals are limited in scope, and therefore possible to accomplish before the next meeting. At the following group meeting, group members discuss how their sub-goals were accomplished, internal and external barriers, and other experiences encountered while attempting to

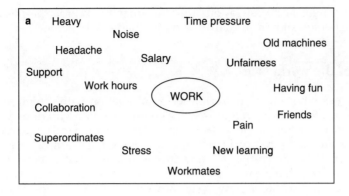

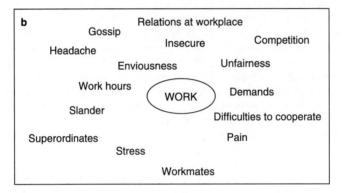

Figure 17.2 *Examples of outcome of the brainstorming session on the theme 'work'. (a) A group with short-term sick leaves only; (b) a group with long-term sick leaves due to musculoskeletal pain*

manage the goal. Experiences and hints are shared within the group, and social support is usually extensive.

When the problem-based approach is adopted, it is important that the worker is allowed to take responsibility not only for determining sub-goals during the rehabilitation process, but also for finding strategies to reach these goals. Workers may have different hindrance factors and different goals for their rehabilitation, and some may need more time than others to obtain their goals. Such differences do not create problems for the group. The source of motivation is intrinsic and built upon a participative approach.

In addition to the problem-based group meetings, employees may choose to participate in other activities, such as physiotherapy, relaxation training, physical activities, stress management and so on. These activities are not mandatory, but are offered as a supplement according to available resources. Over time, they will selectively enrol on the activities they find appropriate for their improvement.

The problem-based method has been applied to groups of workers with pain and diffuse symptoms in the neck and shoulders, but could also be used for other disorders. It is, of course, necessary to go through ordinary medical investigations first, in order to exclude the possibility that the person should primarily undergo medical treatment.

Role of the workplace

Employees who return to work after rehabilitation with a high intrinsic motivation to handle strenuous work conditions and who dare to apply constructive strategies to cope with excessive demands will become 'change agents' in the workplace and provide good examples for others. However, it is uncommon for one single individual at a lower level in the hierarchy to have a realistic chance of accomplishing changes. Rather, it is necessary to take a more system-theoretic view, i.e. supervisors and workmates must also be involved in change processes.

Accordingly, to facilitate the goals of improving work conditions, and also relations and attitudes in the workplace, superordinates or managers of the workers are enrolled in a second group. They meet – at least monthly – to discuss rehabilitation matters and aspects of work, and to get support for a more active approach with regard to workplace changes. The problem-based method is also useful for these groups.

The meetings with superordinates and managers are important arenas for discussions about their difficult roles and responsibilities, in particular with regard to prioritizing between production and employees. A further important goal for the groups is to help and stimulate managers and superordinates to identify problems in their workplace, rather than solely to focus on the individual employee and his or her pain problems. Thereby, rehabilitation and prevention become integrated into one and the same rehabilitation process. Our experiences are that supervisors or managers who are involved from the start of the rehabilitation period will maintain their interest and involvement throughout the period.

Evaluation procedure

Workers suffering from musculoskeletal pain and symptoms were allocated at random to either problem-based rehabilitation or to the rehabilitation normally offered by their OHS units.

It is best for evaluation of any rehabilitation outcome to be directed at the goals of the particular rehabilitation process. In problem-based rehabilitation the predetermined long-term goal is 'to see causes of symptoms and hindrance factors for work, and to change them', i.e. the long-term goal is essentially to start a change process. A positive change process is assumed to promote health via internal and external mediating mechanisms. Accordingly, the measurements used for assessing the rehabilitation outcome focus on the three areas outlined in Figure 17.1 – internal psychosocial resources, conditions at work and self-rated health and quality of life.

The way people assess and evaluate their own health is an interesting endpoint in the evaluation of an intervention, in particular because self-rated health appears to be an important predictor of use of health care

(Bjorner *et al.*, 1996). The SF-36 health questionnaire (Ware and Sherbourne, 1992) is a particularly useful instrument, since it provides measures of physical, mental, social and emotional health. Internal, psychosocial resources are measured by means of two brief instruments on coping (feeling of control) and self-esteem (Pearlin and Schooler, 1978). For measuring conditions at work, use can be made of the questionnaire by Karasek and Theorell (1990). The dimensions of psychological demands, decision latitude at work and social support at work are captured by this instrument.

An evaluation was performed according to the model outlined in Figure 17.3. Self-rated health and quality of life improved more in the problem-based rehabilitation group than among the controls. Those employees who initially had a higher degree of decision latitude and more social support at work showed a more positive improvement in self-rated health over the rehabilitation period. Further, more workers in the problem-based rehabilitation groups improved their self-esteem and coping ability. One way to measure compliance is to note absence and presence at group meetings. In the problem-based groups, workers' presence was found to be extremely high. Also, qualitative information about the social climate in the groups showed social support to be very high.

An important goal of the problem-based rehabilitation process is to change, preferably to improve, essential aspects of the work situation. When measurements are performed before and after rehabilitation only – at an intervening interval of about 4 months – it is not reasonable to expect any major changes yet to have occurred. Rather, changes at work are expected to take place over a longer time period. Tentative results from a one-year follow-up show that problem-based rehabilitation

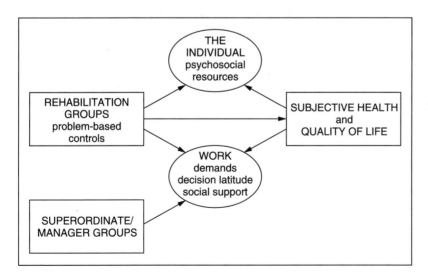

Figure 17.3 *Model for the evaluation process of problem-based rehabilitation*

improves social support at work. In addition, after one year, internal psychosocial resources – self-esteem and coping resources, and self-rated quality of life – were found to have improved more among those who had worked according to the problem-based method.

Concluding remarks

Rehabilitation according to the problem-based method emphasizes the individual's own psychosocial resources as crucial for compliance and for a positive change process. The results highlight the importance of involving the workplace in the rehabilitation process.

References

Barrows, H.S. (1985) *How to Design a Problem-based Curriculum for the Preclinical Years*. Berlin: Springer-Verlag.

Ben-Zira, Z. (1986) Disability, stress and readjustment: the function of the professionals' latent goals and affective behaviour in rehabilitation. *Soc. Sci. Med.*, **23**, 43–55.

Bjorner, J.B., Kristensen, T.S., Orth-Gomér, K., Tibblin, G., Sullivan, M. and Westerholm, P. (eds) (1996) *Self-rated Health, a Useful Concept in Research, Prevention and Clinical Medicine*. Stockholm: Swedish Council for Planning and Coordination of Research (FRN).

Karasek, R. and Theorell, T. (1990) *Healthy Work. Stress, Productivity, and the Reconstruction of Working Life*. New York: Basic Books.

McIntosh, G., Melles, T. and Hall, H. (1995) Guidelines for the identification of barriers to rehabilitation of back injuries. *J. Occup. Rehab.*, **5**, 195–201.

Pearlin, L.I. and Schooler, C. (1978) The structure of coping. *J. Hlth Soc. Behav.*, pp. 19–21.

Ware, J.E. Jr and Sherbourne, C.D. (1992) The MOS 36-item short-form health survey (SF–36). I Conceptual framework and item selection. *Med. Care*, **30**, 473–83.

18

Evaluation courses for OHS professionals

Ewa Menckel, Peter Westerholm and Kaj Husman

On the basis that there is an increasing need for the evaluation of OHS work, there is also a need to train OHS professionals in the use of different models and methods. This chapter concerns two different types of evaluation courses, one international and one national (Sweden). They both offer examples of how courses of this kind might be designed.

The international course was arranged on two occasions, in 1992 and 1997, by the Nordic Institute for Advanced Training in Occupational Health (NIVA). On both occasions, the authors of this chapter, representing Sweden's Institute for Working Life and Finland's Institute of Occupational Health, provided course supervision. The national training course was arranged by the Swedish Institute for Working Life in 1994, and had three course coordinators – a researcher, a senior professional educator of occupational health nurses, and an experienced consultant in work environment and management (also a practising safety engineer) from a Swedish OHS unit.

The international course attracted participants from nine countries, whereas participants on the Swedish course consisted of members of one large OHS organization. The courses had both similarities and differences. They will be described separately below.

International courses on evaluation of OHS

The background to the courses lay in political and social developments, structural changes on labour markets, and the continuous scaling down of public expenditure, leading to an increasing pressure on health services of all kinds to prove their value and to evaluate service outputs. This also applies to OHS.

The first course took place in 1992 (in Finland) and the second in 1997 (in Sweden). Both were of four days in length. The objectives of the courses were formulated as follows. Following attendance, participants should:

• know about current development of methods and approaches in evaluation of health services, in particular OHS;

- be able to apply qualitative and quantitative methods in quality assurance, evaluation and development of their own OHS activities and research.

Target groups were OHS professionals and researchers, and others interested in the evaluation and development of OHS. Most participants were from the Nordic countries, but professionals from the Baltic states and other parts of Europe (Austria, Portugal and the UK) and Asia (India) also attended.

Main topics during both courses were:

- theory of health-services research;
- methods used in evaluation of OHS, with examples and experiences;
- evaluation as a basis for continuing development of OHS;
- quality assurance and evaluation.

The working methods used were lectures, discussions and group work, taking up roughly equal shares of time. Practical issues and case studies from the participants' own experiences – submitted to the faculty in advance of the course – formed the basis for the group discussions.

In comments from the course evaluation, the importance of interaction between faculty and participants was emphasized. The participants rated the balance between theoretical presentations and discussions/group work as excellent or good, and they appreciated the good opportunities for professional contacts between participants and lecturers. The lectures and exercises on evaluation of intervention strategies were of special interest. Alongside impact assessment and qualitative methods, these areas will be given increased emphasis in future courses.

A national evaluation course for OHS staff

There are different ways of learning about evaluation and quality assurance. In the autumn of 1993, the OHS unit responsible for local-government employees in Halland County in Sweden determined to invest in more systematic development work, and regarded the in-house training of 30 or more employees as a suitable point of departure.

The National Institute for Working Life had previously developed a training scheme called 'Evaluation Methodology for Occupational Health Services – quality development in knowledge companies'. The intention was that the Institute's research expertise should be applied in the practical arena. The scheme was regarded as providing an excellent educational foundation for designing a course suiting Halland's needs.

The principal aim of the course was to supply knowledge on evaluation methodology as an element in the quality-assurance work of Halland County OHS. The course was designed to provide a measure of how activities were perceived, and how clients assessed the quality of work performed. Naturally, the course was also intended to generate impulses for change.

The course programme was developed jointly by the Institute and personnel at Halland County OHS. The educational model selected involved performing project work under skilled supervision – a form of 'learning by doing'. This is at heart a participatory and democratic approach, where teaching staff act as advisers rather than relayers of knowledge. It was regarded as essential to a good course outcome that all the OHS unit's personnel were able to take part in the educational process.

The manager of Halland County OHS participated throughout the programme, making for rapid feedback within the organization and direct decision-making on key issues. This was a procedure that added to the impact of the course. Some of the Unit's clients took part in the concluding session to offer their opinions on the evaluation work performed within the framework of the course.

Two course periods

The course was divided into two periods – two days in May 1994, and four days in October 1994. During the time between them, participants worked on various evaluation projects under the guidance of the course coordinators.

During the first course period the aims and contents of the course were presented. Participants were offered a review of theoretical frameworks for evaluation and quality assurance. Preparations were made for the individual projects.

At first, there was a degree of uncertainty over the aims of the course and the extent of the project work involved. But even by the first evening, participants had become highly involved in discussing conceivable subjects and possible collaborating partners. Project groups were formed at the initiative of the participants. Many of them found a suitable point of departure in a specific problem they had encountered in everyday working life.

After the second day, a brief course evaluation was performed. It proved that the greatest merit so far had been to increase understanding of what evaluation is and what quality assurance entails in practice. The group discussions were regarded as valuable, and the project work as stimulating. The training had provided participants with insights into how they could develop in their work.

In principle, the course coordinators had two approaches to choose between during the course. There was the possibility of working in a traditional manner, giving formal approval to project designs and methods, instruments and reports. Or, they could adopt a more open attitude, where participants could themselves seek knowledge and support according to the needs that developed during the evaluation process. In practice, it was a simple choice to make. The participants largely preferred to work freely and select their own evaluation methods.

Key aspects of course design are summarized under the points below. The course:

- was offered to a united working group;
- was provided simultaneously to all personnel in the OHS unit;
- took its point of departure in prevailing local conditions;
- was based on all participants having to make an active effort;
- was needed to develop the Unit's operations;
- was designed to work for change as a natural part of the Unit's activities.

Interactive training and supervision

The time between the introductory and concluding parts of the course – the project period – was a period of interactive training and supervised work (see Figure 18.1). The period was introduced with a general review of the relevant literature. Preliminary project plans were handed over to the course coordinators – containing a statement of problem addressed, a description of selected methods, and sometimes a proposal for items to be included on a survey (questionnaire) instrument of some kind.

The supervisors responded to each plan on the telephone, and also sent an encouraging letter to all participants with questions designed to stimulate the project work and to give some general pieces of advice on implementation. More concrete advice was given in specific cases.

The participants were eager to start their projects prior to their forthcoming vacation. The projects covered a very wide range of OHS activities. A variety of programmes and activities were scrutinized, as too was the in-house efficiency of OHS. The evaluations offered opportu-

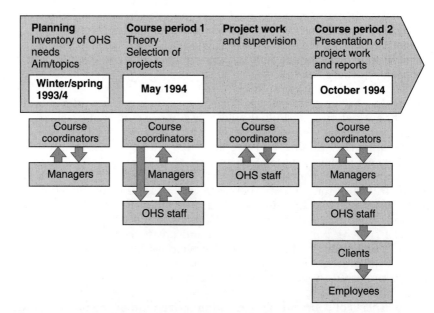

Figure 18.1 *Interactive planning and implementation of the OHS evaluation course*

nities to penetrate different issues thoroughly, and to generate problem solutions.

Supervision was provided throughout the course period. Some of the participants had difficulties in contacting their envisaged study group/interviewees. Staffing changes at the Unit during the course affected the composition of some project groups. However, all 15 projects were completed and documented in good time before the concluding course days (see Table 18.1).

For these days, the participants were divided into two groups on the basis of workplace. The days – two per group – were principally

Table 18.1 *Fifteen projects designed by OHS staff to enhance work quality and efficiency*

Project title and main topics	Evaluator	Methods
1 A chemical products database: good protection against harmful substances?	Two safety engineers	Questionnaires to 44 clients
2 Steering team: an efficient method for information?	Senior physician	Interviews with 20 managers
3 OHS-awareness at executive level?	Site manager	Open questions to 12 principal clients
4 The safety engineer: a key link in the environmental arena?	Two safety engineers	Discussions with and questionnaires to 8 managers
5 Problems related to sick buildings: who is responsible for what, and when?	Physician, safety engineer, and nurse	Interviews with all involved
6 Alternative interviews: a faster way of getting results?	Physician	Questionnaire to supervisors and safety representatives
7 Computerized workplaces: education improves the work environment?	Nurse	Interviews and observations in the workplace
8 Job transfers: training counteracts stress injuries?	Two physiotherapists and a nurse	Questionnaires to 18 participants
9 Crisis experiences: study circles counteract burn-out?	Social psychologist	Questionnaires to 28 ambulance drivers
10 Individual re-adaptation: contact person is important?	Senior physician	Questionnaires to and interviews with 22 clinic and ward managers
11 Rehabilitation in groups: positive for all parties?	Physiotherapist and nurse	Interviews with and questionnaires to 23 employees and managers
12 The keep-fit representative: support and stimulation at work?	Three physical welfare officers	Interviews at three wards
13 Sequential training: efficient physical welfare services and rehabilitation?	Nurse	Questionnaire to 50 employees
14 Improved time sheets: statistics and methods	Two clerical officers	Interviews with all OHS staff
15 Good OHS service? Scrutiny of health aspects	Administrative manager, two clerical officers and nurse	Questions to 85 employees

devoted to exchanges of experiences related to the project reports. Theoretical aspects were tailored to the needs that emerged on review. A lecture on ethical aspects of OHS work proved to be particularly important.

Participants provided a summary report of their evaluation. An 'opponent' group, appointed by the course coordinators, then introduced a discussion in each case. The course coordinators and the manager of the OHS provided analytic inputs, proposed improvements and suggested ideas for follow-up. On four occasions, the OHS client concerned was also present. This gave the reports further roots in reality, and provided deeper insight into clients' needs.

Summary of experiences and concluding remarks

The project discussions provided the basis for many work improvements at the OHS unit. Several new project groups were formed to further develop work in a process of change. It was not unusual for participants to be startled by the realization of a new aspect or perspective. They also received a strong reminder of the collective expertise residing in OHS.

The course and the fifteen projects are documented in a published report entitled 'Evaluate – quality development in Occupational Health Services') (Menckel *et al.*, 1995, in Swedish). It is now used by the OHS as a marketing report to customers and others.

Reference

Menckel, E., Ekeberg, C., Österblom, L. and Fahlstedt, P. (1995) *Utvärdera – kvalitetsutveckling i företagshälsovård*. The Swedish Institute of Occupational Health, Stockholm.

Part 3
PERSPECTIVES AND FUTURE TRENDS

19

Evaluation and ethics in an OHS setting

Peter Westerholm

Ethics, in the context of this book, imply a reference to the principles of right conduct or practice in evaluating occupational health practices. What particular difficulties do evaluators in this field face? What violations of ethical principles may occur? An overview is given of the basic principles involved, and reference is made to some professional guidelines in current use. Practical guidance is provided on including agreements on ethically sensitive issues in evaluation contracts, and attention is drawn to some pitfalls to avoid in observing ethical conduct in evaluations.

Good ethics – what is it?

Ethics are fundamentally related to human action. They concern what one does or does not do, and also how it is done. An action undertaken may affect others in a desirable, intended way, or – conversely – in a way that is undesired or unintended. Further, what is a desirable outcome or consequence for some stakeholders may not be regarded as such by others. Evaluators hold special powers in that their judgements may lead to improvements in practices, but may also injure the self-esteem, reputation and career prospects of either those evaluated, other parties involved in the evaluation, or both. In planning and conducting an evaluation, it is therefore essential to bear in mind the values to be safeguarded. The ethical issues of evaluation practice are in many respects the same as those of social research in general.

The following value criteria are often referred to as basic principles for good ethics in social and health research:

- beneficence;
- non-maleficence;
- respecting autonomy;
- justice.

Beneficence means avoiding unnecessary harm and maximizing good outcomes. This entails that the evaluation is valid, that evaluators are competent and characterized by professional conduct of high standards, that stakeholders are fully informed, and that results are disseminated to all concerned. In a general and global sense, it implies the doing of good deeds to everyone concerned, including those evaluated – whether the latter consist of professional groups, health-service programmes or organizations, the sponsors of the evaluation, or other interested parties.

Non-maleficence is, practically speaking, a clarification of the benefi-cence criterion. It implies the principle of not doing harm.

Respect means considering the autonomy and integrity of persons, groups and organizations whose practices are being assessed, and strictly observing principles of informal voluntary consent and the safe-guarding of confidential information. Respect also includes the princi-ples of non-coercion and non-manipulation.

Coercion, implying the use of force or threats to secure compliance or access to information, is clearly not consistent with good evaluation practice. In actual practice this is not, however, a common problem. Non-manipulation is an equally important principle, since manipulation may be insidious. Subjects under evaluation are not always aware of the full implications of the underlying motives, initiation, carrying-out and use of an evaluation, and what consequences these may have for them person-ally. This is what makes the principle of informed consent an essential basis of ethics in evaluations. Informed consent means that the persons who agree to participate understand the evaluation project – including its aims, their own role in it, and what the information will be used for.

Justice means equitable and fair treatment – and representation – of the stakeholders involved – in all the planning and performance steps an evaluation involves.

Propriety

Ethics in evaluation are closely related to what are sometimes referred to as propriety standards. The United States Joint Committee on Standards for Educational Evaluation (1994) has provided the following summary of the objectives of its propriety standards:

> The propriety standards are intended to ensure that an evaluation will be conducted legally, ethically and with due regard for the welfare of those involved in the evaluation, as well as those affected by its results. These standards are as follows:
>
> - **P1 Service Orientation:** Evaluations should be designed to assist organizations to address and effectively serve the needs of the full range of targeted participants.
> - **P2 Formal Agreements:** Obligations of the formal parties to an evaluation (what is to be done, how, by whom, when) should be agreed in writing, so that these parties are obligated to adhere to all conditions of the agreement or formally to renegotiate it.
> - **P3 Rights of Human Subjects:** Evaluations should be designed and conducted to respect and protect the rights and welfare of human subjects.
> - **P4 Human Interactions:** Evaluators should respect human dignity

and worth in their interactions with persons associated with an evaluation, so that participants are not threatened or harmed.

- **P5 Complete and Fair Assessment:** The evaluation should be complete and fair in its examination and recording of strengths and weaknesses of the programme being evaluated, so that strengths can be built upon and problem areas addressed.
- **P6 Disclosure of Findings:** The formal parties to an evaluation should ensure that the full set of evaluation findings along with pertinent limitations are made accessible to the persons affected by the evaluation, and any others with expressed legal rights to receive the results.
- **P7 Conflict of Interest:** Conflict of interest should be dealt with openly and honestly, so that it does not compromise the evaluation processes and results.
- **P8 Fiscal Responsibility:** The evaluator's allocation and expenditure of resources should reflect sound accountability procedure and otherwise be prudent and ethically responsible, so that expenditures are accounted for and appropriate.

Confidentiality

Confidentiality is one of the fundamental issues in evaluations. An evaluator is privy to information on companies, enterprise departments, OHS units, the populations served by the units, managements of companies and occupational health professionals, and many other categories of staff. This information may be – in itself or in aggregate forms – sensitive to the integrity of the persons, groups or organizations involved. It may become available to unauthorized persons, and it may be used for purposes and ways which are adverse to those who have supplied it.

Some types of information are company-confidential. Other types, such as health information on individuals, may be confidential at individual subject level. In evaluations, the confidentiality of information must constantly be borne in mind. This basically applies to all kinds of evaluations, including second or third party evaluations.

It is a hallmark of professionalism of evaluators to be aware of the confidentiality issues arising during the process, to be aware of obligations to stakeholders, and to have a constant awareness of the arena in which the evaluation is taking place. A necessary precondition for gaining and maintaining access, cooperation and trust is to agree and make explicit how information gathered for the evaluation will be reported and made available. In second and third party evaluations, access to – say – patient records and other health service documents that are not public needs to be discussed at the planning stage with the sponsors of the evaluation. Restrictions on access to and use of such records may limit the scope of the evaluation and have implications for its design.

Confidentiality issues arise in interviews with representatives of companies and populations served by OHS, occupational health professionals and others. In collection of such information, it is necessary to have a clear understanding of the confidentiality rules that apply. In evaluation agreements, it should be stated how the collected information will be used and disseminated, and whether information provided will be attributed to recognizable individuals or made available to persons or groups not participating in the interviews.

Who needs to be informed?

Matters of the public or private status of the final evaluation report and publication rights should also be agreed upon with the sponsor and the OHS units involved at the beginning of any evaluation. There will often be many people wanting to know what the evaluator found out. It is also necessary to agree on who will make the report available, and what the evaluators can and cannot say – in either public or informal settings – during and after the evaluation (see Øvretveit, 1998). Many problems and misunderstandings can be prevented by including evaluation contract clauses on responsibilities and agreements with regard to confidentiality and right to information.

The status and handling of the final evaluation report, including publication rights, should be agreed during the planning of an evaluation. It often happens that groups and persons outside the arena of a particular evaluation want to find out about its results. They may request copies of the evaluation report. The principles in handling such requests need to be settled and agreed in advance.

An evaluator acting ethically will give high priority to the communication phase when the results of the evaluation are made available. Sponsors and users of an evaluation have invested funding and resources for the evaluation to be carried out. They may have expectations and notions about the use of the evaluation report and its potential to improve conditions in the workplace. The evaluator has a moral duty to communicate the findings and conclusions of the evaluation, and also to ascertain that the results of the evaluation are correctly understood and not misinterpreted. Ethical conduct on the part of an evaluator also includes an obligation to assist sponsors and the OHS evaluated to explore the implications of his/her findings with a view to improving OHS practices and performance (see Øvretveit, 1998).

Many research institutions and social research bodies have adopted codes of ethics that provide a good basis for evaluations of policies and practices in the field of occupational health.

The ethical code of practice of the British Social Resource Association of the UK is one such example. The earlier mentioned US Program Evaluation Standards adopted by the Joint Committee on Standards for Educational Evaluation (1994) is another. Recently, the Canadian Evaluation Society (1996) has published guidelines for ethical conduct of evaluators. These guidelines are based on the three principal criteria of **competence**, **integrity** and **accountability** as follows.

1 **Competence:** Evaluators are to be competent in their provision of service.

   1.1 Evaluators should apply systematic methods of enquiry appropriate to the evaluation.

   1.2 Evaluators should possess or provide content knowledge appropriate for the evaluation.

   1.3 Evaluators should continuously strive to improve their methodological and practice skills.

2 **Integrity:** Evaluators are to act with integrity in their relationship with all stakeholders.

   2.1 Evaluators should accurately represent their level of skills and knowledge.

   2.2 Evaluators should declare any conflict of interest to clients before embarking on an evaluation project and at any point where such conflict occurs. This includes conflict of interest on the part of either evaluator or stakeholder.

   2.3 Evaluators should be sensitive to the cultural and social environment of all stakeholders and conduct themselves in a manner appropriate to this environment.

   2.4 Evaluators should confer with the client on contractual decisions such as confidentiality, privacy, communication and ownership of finding and reports.

3 **Accountability:** Evaluators are to be accountable for their performance and their product.

   3.1 Evaluators should be responsible for the provision of information to clients to facilitate their decision-making concerning the selection of appropriate evaluation strategies and methodologies. Such information should include the limitations of selected methodology.

   3.2 Evaluators should be responsible for the clear, accurate and fair, written and/or oral presentation of study findings and limitations, and recommendations.

   3.3 Evaluators should be responsible in their fiscal decision-making so that expenditures are accounted for and clients receive good value for their dollars.

   3.4 Evaluators should be responsible for the completion of the evaluation within a reasonable time as agreed to with the clients. Such agreements should acknowledge unprecedented delays resulting from factors beyond the evaluator's control.

Common errors

A number of errors are commonly made in evaluation practice:

- To assume that doing whatever the client or the sponsor wants or whatever is judged to benefit the sponsor is ethically correct. In an ethical perspective the client is simply not always right.
- To regard the managers of programmes as sole beneficiaries of an evaluation. It may be all too easy to pay less attention to the needs of

other important stakeholders. This is actually one of the fundamental difficulties or dilemmas in an internal evaluation of a service programme. How are the needs of clients or the populations served taken properly into account when focusing the evaluation entirely on the needs of the organization?

- The belief that the written evaluation contract is to be followed to the letter whatever new or unexpected findings may come up during the evaluation process. It may occur, for example, that the evaluator observes serious human rights abuse in an occupational health programme not encompassed by the evaluation contract. To follow the contract may be formally the correct decision. It does not, however, absolve the evaluator from the moral responsibility to react.
- The belief that the use of a method in the health services which is validated as a research tool guarantees ethically sound practice in occupational health. In, for example, the practices of drug testing in the workplace – implying compulsory examinations of urine specimens of employed staff for traces of narcotic drugs – the analytical methods used for examination may be of high-grade validity. From this does not follow, however, that their implementation in practice is warranted and ethically sound. Are the tests needed at all?
- The notion that the evaluator's responsibility is to collect information from all stakeholders and accept everyone's opinion equally. There is an ethical obligation for the evaluator to listen to the views of everyone concerned but not to accept all views as morally equal.
- The disregard or neglect of important stakeholders who do not have the powers or opportunities to contribute with their experiences and views in the evaluation. There is a moral responsibility for the evaluator to include the interests of all. Ethical conduct on the part of an evaluator implies the assumption of the role of guardian of democratic values.

For further discussion of traps to be avoided by the ethically conscious evaluator, see House (1994).

The evaluation of OHS programmes or activities means assessment of professionals, professional organizations and their actions. This is a challenging task to the evaluator – since one of the aspects which cannot, and indeed should not, be avoided is evaluation of the ethical standards of conduct of those being evaluated. This is a matter of reconciling the professional ethics of the evaluator with the professional ethics of the OHS under evaluation. The following questions apply to both the evaluator and those evaluated:

- Is it ethical to market and provide service for which you are not capable or competent?
- Is it ethical to provide services in which you do not have confidence?
- Is it ethical to provide services not needed by the customer or client?
- Is it ethical to market and provide services primarily designed to preserve one's own professional power base?

In many countries there is an increasing practice by OHS organizations to include clauses or statements on ethics in quality manuals, procedure guidelines, mission statements and other documents used in management of the organization and its activities. In evaluating such documents and their implementation it is important to recognize that the outcome of the evaluation is to a significant degree dependent on both the value sets of those evaluated and those of the evaluator. Keeping this in mind, however, the principles of conducting an evaluation apply. This means that the first step is to examine the documents of the OHS organization being evaluated where the ethical norms or principles are elaborated. Issues and operations deserving close examination are:

- Role and task of the organization and the occupational health professionals.
- Professional integrity, impartiality and independence.
- Information and communication on health hazard assessments.
- Information and communication on results of health surveillance staff.
- Protection and safeguarding of confidential information on the enterprise itself and on the health of staff members.
- Clauses on ethics in employment contracts for OH professionals.
- Reference to professional ethical codes of OH professionals.

In a second stage, following the review of documents, the observations made are followed up with a view to examining implementation of ethical principles or guidelines.

For a discussion of issues arising at the interface between professional *ethos* and duties to customers and demands in markets, see Griffiths and Lucas (1996).

For over-riding ethical principles in OHS, the reader is referred to the Ethical Guidelines for Occupational Health Professionals issued by the International Commission on Occupational Health (ICOH, 1992).

The application of ethical principles to the actual conduct of an evaluation may be a very demanding task. Ethical principles are abstract, and it is not always obvious how they should be applied in concrete situations. The practice of evaluating health services – including OHS – implies that the evaluator is confronted with a range of action-related and practical issues. The first question to ask should perhaps not be 'What are the ethical issues of evaluations?' It may be more helpful to ask 'Which issues in this evaluation are ethical?' The ethical issues concern the actions planned and undertaken, and in what ways their underlying motives involve the value criteria of beneficence, non-maleficence, respect, and justice. They also include examinations of health practices to which competing, or even conflicting, values apply.

Ethics in the field of evaluation, and evaluation of human service organizations (such as OHS) in particular, may be very demanding. The balancing of the value principles of ethics in concrete evaluations of such organizations is a fundamental challenge to the professionalism and probity of the evaluator. Some guidance on ethical conduct of the evaluator in a self-assessment may be provided by questions such as:

- Have I been fair and balanced in my assessment of the interest of all stakeholders – including both short-term and longer-term interests – in examining this OHS organization or programme?

- What are my feelings when looking into the mirror and seeing my own reflection?
- How would my family and friends – including my professional colleagues – value my performance if it became known to them how I have carried out this evaluation?
- What would I feel like if my performance became publicly known and was referred to in the media?

These elementary questions reflect the fact that professional ethics and professional ethical conduct deal, in a fundamental way, with the issues of raising a person's own values to a conscious level of perception and thinking.

A prerequisite for gaining access to information and the trust of stakeholders is to agree in advance – and make explicit to sponsors and other interested parties – how information collected will be used and made available in reporting an evaluation. It is often advisable to prepare a statement on confidentiality rules for implementation in the examination of documents, the conduct of interviews, and the use of other sources of information.

An elementary test to make in considering ethical implications of an action is to consider each alternative by asking ourselves 'How would I defend this particular option if required to do so before a broad audience?' (see Cooper, 1998).

The evaluation contract

Many of the ethical and other problems in an evaluation can be avoided by drawing up a contract defining responsibilities and agreement on matters pertinent to good ethical standards.

A prerequisite for gaining access to information and the trust of stakeholders is to agree in advance – and make explicit to sponsors and other interested parties – how information collected will be used and made available in reporting an evaluation. It is often advisable to prepare a statement on confidentiality rules for implementation in the examination of documents, the conduct of interviews and the use of other sources of information.

The status and handling of the final evaluation report, including publication rights, should be agreed during the planning of an evaluation. It often happens that groups and persons outside the arena of the evaluation want to find out about the results of the evaluation. They may request copies of the evaluation report. The principles in handling such requests need to be settled and agreed in advance.

This does not detract from the ethical obligation of the evaluator to communicate results to sponsors and users of the evaluation. But it entails a moral duty to ascertain that the results of an evaluation and its report are correctly understood, and also an obligation to assist in exploring the implications of evaluation findings with a view to improving OHS practices.

References

Cooper, T. (1998) *The Responsible Administrator*. San Francisco: Jossey–Bass.
Griffiths, M.R. and Lucas, J.R. (1996) *Ethical Economics*. London: Macmillan.
Health Communication Unit (1998) *Evaluating Health Promotion Programmes*. Centre for Health Protection, University of Toronto.
House, E. (1994) *Professional Evaluation*. Newbury Park, CA: Sage Publications.
International Commission on Occupational Health (ICOH) (1992) *International Code of Ethics for Occupational Health Professionals*. Geneva: International Commission on Occupational Health/International Labour Office.
Joint Committee on Standards for Educational Evaluation (Chair: James R. Sanders) (1994) *Standards for Educational Evaluation*. Thousand Oaks ,CA: Sage Publications.
Øvretveit, J. (1998) *Evaluating Health Interventions*. Milton Keynes: Open University Press.

20

Economic appraisal in occupational health

Jorma Rantanen

The advantages and shortcomings of economic appraisals of occupational health services (OHS) are discussed in some detail. Broadly, economic analyses break down into cost–benefit analyses (CBAs) and various forms of cost-effectiveness analyses (CEAs). Recently, both human resource analysis and ethical values have been incorporated into assessment procedures. The author adopts a generally favourable stance on economic appraisal of OHS, but stresses the need to bear in mind its intrinsic limitations and the need for further methodological development. How to incorporate human values is an issue of particular importance.

Shortcomings of economic analyses in OH

Economic analysis of services and activities carried out in the public sector have obtained a very prominent position in present market-oriented societies – not only in discussions and decisions on issues that directly involve economic aspects, but also in choices of social priorities, including those concerning health care (Rantanen, 1997).

While hundreds of research projects have been initiated for the economic analysis of health services, the people interested in ethical and value systems in the health sector have expressed concern about unethical economization in the sector (which originally was aimed to serve exclusively human values). Besides present 'ideological' reasons, economic appraisal has become relevant to the prioritization of actions in the health care arena, and also to the demonstration of economic efficiency in the health sector.

On the other hand, economic analysis of loss caused by various health problems is used as an argument for justifying the existence of activities for prevention, control and treatment, and also for identifying targets and priorities for research and practical actions (Box 20.1). Again, warning voices have been raised concerning the bias that may occur in looking at economy only, and not the ability of health programmes to produce health, quality of life and well-being (Westerholm, 1996).

Box 20.1 Justification for measuring burden of disease and injury (Murray and Lopez, 1994)

1 Can aid priority setting for health services.
2 Can direct research priorities.
3 Can identify disadvantaged groups for interventions.
4 Can provide comparable measure for intervention, programme and sector evaluation and planning.

Analysis of cost can be performed at various levels of the system, starting from global and ending at individual or family level. The level at which any analysis is made may substantially affect its outcome – due to numerous and often complicated transfers of costs and benefits from one level to another. The most common of such transfers is the shift in costs from private enterprise to the national economy, which has been regarded as a problem in many countries.

A probable bias is over-estimation of the cost-effectiveness of the private sector, which is selective in choosing only services that are profitable. It limits service provision to densely populated areas, and only provides service at hours when people are most active. In this context, the public sector may appear less effective, given its obligation to carry out universal service provision and 24-hour service.

In the course of integrating economies, the transfer of costs may become even more complicated due to numerous cross-border transactions. Development aid programmes contribute either to the compensation of losses or to the prevention of impairments. The European Union, with its numerous subsidizing systems, is a good example of this kind of complexity. Accordingly, any final and precise answer to the question of what the costs of work-related health impairments actually are is difficult to give.

Methods still in need of development

Most studies concerned with the economic analysis of health programmes warn about the wide margin of errors to which insufficient methodologies give rise. Inaccuracy in the economic analysis of occupational injuries and diseases has, for example, been attributed to poor coverage and weak efficiency of registration of occupationally related health problems.

Due to such weaknesses, international comparisons are not very useful. There are also numerous other sources of error, e.g. the variation in social security and compensation principles between different countries and differences in the coverage of various populations by insurance, in compensation of impaired health, and in the definitions of injury and disease.

The outcome of any analysis also depends substantially on the method used for calculation. For example, how health care and social security costs are calculated, and how loss of production is estimated are still

Table 20.1 *Methods for calculating burden of disease and injury*

Type of analysis	Measure of value
Monetary based	
Human capital (Koopmanschap, 1994)	Present discounted value of person's income stream
Friction cost (Koopmanschap, 1994)	Costs to the society and enterprise from loss of work input and production until the loss is replaced
Wage-risk analysis (Hammer, 1997)	Analysis of wage differences between safe and risky but otherwise comparable occupations
Willingness to pay (Hammer, 1997)	Individuals' willingness to pay for prevention of negative health outcome
Productivity model (Ahonen, 1995)	Comparison of investments to health with short-term benefits in loss control and productivity gains
Health based	
Quality Adjusted Life Years (QUALY) (Barnum, 1987)	Interviewed respondents interest to trade off certain type of health problem against other types of health problem
Disability Adjusted Life Years (DALY) (Murray and Lopez, 1994)	Weighted valuation and comparison of death and disability at different ages

Table 20.2 *Main approaches in economic appraisal*

Characteristics	Cost–benefit analysis (C/B)	Cost–efficacy analysis (C/E)	Cost-effectiveness analysis (C/EE)
Basic orientation	Economic, operative	Technical, operative	Health values
Sensitivity	Low	High	High
Specificity	High	High	Low
Indicators	Money	Outputs	Achieved goals
Application areas	Wide	Limited	Limited
Applicable to health programmes	Poorly	Well	Well
Comparative	Yes	Yes	No or poorly

major analytic problems. Are, for example, the payroll expenses of health-service personnel 'costs', or are they 'products' that should be counted as part of GNP?

There are two main approaches to the analysis of the burden of diseases and injuries – cost–benefit analysis and cost–effectiveness analysis. The most important characteristics of methods currently in use are described in Table 20.1, and a comparison between them in relation to analysis of health programmes is presented in Table 20.2.

Cost–benefit analysis

In addition to the aspects referred to in Table 20.2, cost–benefit analysis (CBA) has a number of strengths and weaknesses. Its main advantage is that problems have just one measure, i.e. in terms of money. But there are also numerous drawbacks:

- costs are usually tangible and measurable, whereas benefits are abstract and difficult to measure;
- costs are incurred immediately or in a measurable period of time, whereas benefits may show considerable latency;
- costs are well definable conceptually, whereas benefits may be valued differently according to evaluator;
- costs and benefits may accrue to different actors (due to the transfers mentioned above);
- valuing human health, disease or life economically involves a number of ethical issues, which are difficult to solve.

The most recently developed CBAs are based on friction cost calculation (Koopmanchap, 1994) and productivity analysis (Ahonen and Luopajärvi, 1996). In the health arena, the former calculates the disturbances for company or society entailed by health impairment of the worker, while the latter analyses return times for investments made for health programmes.

In particular, the friction cost method is sensitive to factors in the societal macro system. If, for example, there is a surplus of labour, the cost of replacement of injured or diseased workers is lower than in times of universal shortage of labour. Further, monetarization of human health has been criticized by ethicists. No satisfactory solutions to this problem have so far been found.

Cost-effectiveness analysis

Cost-effectiveness analyses (CEA) do not provide any direct answers concerning costs or benefits of a health programme or problem, but can be used for ranking different health problems or programmes for the purpose of health policy-making. Again, a number of strengths and weaknesses of the method can be indicated:

- the CEA model is based on comparison of health values;
- comparison of different types of ill-health or injury is difficult;
- effectiveness in solution of a problem does not necessarily reflect the priority position of the problem in terms of health needs;
- subjectively, for each individual, his or her health problem is of the utmost importance regardless of its social ranking.

Some recently developed methods are based on Disability Adjusted Life Years (DALYs) (see Murray and Lopez, 1994). Key indicators of the burden of disease are developed by combining both mortality and morbidity. The method considers value of time lived at different ages (comparing time lived as disabled with time lost by premature mortality), and also includes a modest percentage discount (3%) into the future. In fact, the DALY method calculates losses by risk factor, by disease and by consequence. Much caution needs still to be exercised in the use of

DALYs due to problems in setting values for the life of, for example, different age groups.

Scientific discussion has generated criticism of both the CBA and CEA methods. The core of the criticism focuses on difficulties in evaluating health and life at various ages, and in setting the rate at which current health problems should be discounted into the future. Nevertheless, new methods have no doubt substantially improved analytic opportunities for the measurement of the cost and health burden of diseases and injuries.

A third new approach, introduced recently in the Nordic countries and in The Netherlands, consists in the preparation of a so-called social report – of an enterprise, sector of the economy, or a nation. This is an approach that integrates the analysis of costs and benefits with the development and management of human resources from economic, social and ethical perspectives (Aronsson et al., 1994). Such a human-resource-development approach has the merit of considering the value of human resources to the company.

Global burden of occupational injuries and diseases

Due to the poor registration of occupational accidents in about 60% of the UN member countries and to the great variation in registration practices between countries, accurate global estimates for accidents are difficult to give.

Even where statistics are available, a registration paradox is likely to arise. The countries with the highest standard of occupational safety and health also show the highest accident and disease rates due to the facts that such countries also have the best registration procedures and the widest conceptual coverage of registered outcomes.

Differences in recorded numbers vary widely, e.g. because some countries register only accidents that occur in the workplace and lead to sickness absence of three or more days. By contrast, Finland and Sweden, for example, register all accidents that take place either on the work site, in traffic occupations, or during commuting (to and from work). All employed and self-employed persons are covered, and all company sizes included. Some other countries do not register commuting accidents; the self-employed and small-scale industries may also remain uncovered, and the concept of accident may be highly exclusive. Such differences in the definition of accidents and in registration practice may give rise to major discrepancies in accident rates, and consequently in cost estimates.

Sets of global estimates are available for both occupational accidents and occupational diseases. The WHO experts (Murray and Lopez, 1994) estimated global disease burdens using estimated Disability Adjusted Life Years (DALYs) as a measure. They obtained, for the two main regions of the world, a total disease and injury burden of 1360 billion DALYs. About 363 billion DALYs (27%) were estimated to be lost by the population at working age, and about 300–550 million from direct occupational causes; 3.4 million DALYs are attributed to occupational injuries and 137 000 to fatalities.

Table 20.3 *Global burden of the most important occupational diseases and injuries, 1990*

	Burden (10^6 DALYs)
Neuropsychiatric	93
Injuries[a]	81
Cancer	79
Chronic respiratory	47
Musculoskeletal	18
Total	318

[a]Including accidents, fires, poisonings, falls etc.
Source: World Development Report, 1993

The share of occupational cancer in total DALYs can also be estimated, as too the burden of the top five occupational diseases (World Development Report, 1993) (see Table 20.3).

An independent calculation by Dr Mikheev of WHO, made on the basis of data on occupational diseases from a few model countries and founded on accident statistics of the ILO, includes some 68–157 million occupational diseases (average 112.5 million) (WHO, 1995) and 125 million occupational accidents (of which 225 000 were fatal).

Using Nordic statistics as a starting point, the estimate places the total cost of occupational diseases and accidents in the world at no less than US$ 900 billion per year, i.e. at US$ 375 per member of the workforce. It is paradoxical that the countries with the smallest economic resources, and the least resources for compensation of the consequences of accidents and diseases, have the highest burdens in terms of these outcomes. Most employers, and even many governments, are not yet able to carry out cost–benefit or cost-effectiveness analyses, and this may lead to the under-prioritization of occupational health.

Burden to national economy

There are only weakly systematic data for the economic analysis of costs of occupational injuries at national level. One of the most comprehensive studies was conducted in the Nordic countries – by calculating economic loss in relation to nine major outcomes, including diseases, accidents and fatalities (Hansen, 1993).

The method employed was so-called 'cost-of-illness' calculation, including assessment of health care costs, costs of early retirement, and costs of premature mortality. The study estimated work-related fractions of total morbidity among the working population, and – by using national statistics – estimated burden of care, loss of productive working time, and cost of pensions.

The estimated total cost of diseases is 15–22% of GNP. For work-related causes, the loss varied by country – in the range 1.5% to 5% of GNP. The greatest loss was attributable to musculoskeletal diseases, respiratory disorders, cardiovascular diseases, and accidents – which jointly accounted for about 50%. In the USA, the costs of occupational accidents in 1994 were about US$ 121 billion – about 2% of GDP, and US$ 1000/capita in the workforce (NIOSH, 1994).

In Sweden, the total economic loss sustained from accidents of any kind was US$ 6.2 billion (about 3% of GDP), and the directly work-related fraction was about 50%. This amounts to a cost of about US$ 689/capita in the workforce (Jansson and Springfeldt, 1996). This calculation of burden was made using the production–loss method, which includes the following parameters:

A. Human losses
  • short-term absence
  • long-term absence
  • permanent impairment
  • fatality
B. Production losses
  • quality deterioration
  • production loss
  • intrinsic cost of absence
  • follow-up and relocation
  • administration
  • follow-up of counter-measures

As well as analyses of accidents and occupational diseases, analysis of the financial consequences of occupational stress-related disorders has been performed at national level in both Sweden and in Denmark (Levi and Lunde-Jensen, 1996). In Sweden, stress-related disorders (mainly cardiovascular) were found to account for 10% of all costs of work-related illness.

In Denmark, a detailed economic analysis of total, and also stress-associated, work-related illnesses has been performed. A figure of 2.5% of GDP was found for total work-related illness, and one of 0.1% of GDP for stress-related outcomes (Levi and Lunde-Jensen, 1996).

To sum up, while total costs of directly occupational plus work-related health outcomes amount to about 10% of GNP (range 5–10), a roughly equal cost is sustained as a result of loss of work input – due to life years lost, or loss of work capacity. Reduction in such loss would entail a substantial growth in productivity, contribute to improved quality of life for workers, and also better quality of products.

Costs at workplace level

The ultimate decisions on health and safety are made at company level. This is why it is important to analyse the costs of accidents and diseases also for individual companies. Numerous models for such analysis are available. They calculate the burden of both occupational and non-occupational morbidity, and also the impact of occupational accidents on a company's finances.

Both direct (visible) and indirect (hidden) costs can be estimated. Some authors have proposed ratios of as high as 1:4 between direct and indirect costs. Both categories may vary substantially between companies. It is self-evident, for example, that rates of work-related diseases and injuries may vary considerably by company and sector of the economy (e.g. between services and manufacturing).

Surprisingly, there is also much variation between individual companies in the same sector of industry, and even between companies of the same size category. Variations as great as two- to four-fold have been detected in accident rates between otherwise comparable enterprises (Aaltonen, 1996). In addition to variation in accident and disease rates, there is also considerable cost variation due to the differential impacts injuries have on production.

The cost of occupational accidents and diseases out of the total turnover of a company has ranged in Finland from 0.1 to over 1%. Accident-insurance compensations alone may amount to 0.8% of turnover. For example, total economic loss from accidents in Nordic furniture industries varied between 0.2% (Sweden) to 0.5% (Finland) of the total wages paid by the companies concerned.

Not only accidents and occupational diseases but also work-related stress have been assessed for costs (Cooper *et al.*, 1996). The costs of stress-related health impairments were measured principally in the form of sickness absenteeism, loss of productivity, and social-security expenses.

Stress-prevention programmes in Sweden have been found to result in a 12% reduction in production costs, with interventions being covered by their own costs. In The Netherlands, similar interventions have been found to be clearly positive in cost–benefit terms, sickness absenteeism being reduced by 30% (of which one third was directly attributed to the interventions). There is also a UK example showing a clear qualitative improvement in health indicators, though cost–benefit analysis was not performed.

A new computerized system (called 'TERVUS') for the assessment of occupational health and safety costs and benefits from OHS programmes has been developed by the Finnish Institute of Occupational Health (Ahonen and Luopajärvi, 1996). The software guides accurate registration and calculation of both investments in and outputs of a programme, and also displays pay-back times as calculation outcomes.

Numerous cases of occupational health and safety interventions have been analysed, and the pay-back times of interventions (most often less than one year) have often been found to be surprisingly low. The software, in addition to providing a technical tool for cost–benefit analysis, also creates awareness of usability and demonstrates advantages of occupational health to company productivity. The software is designed for use even by analysts who do not have competence in cost–benefit analysis (personnel managers in companies, OHS personnel, etc.).

Future perspectives

Constriction of resources and political changes have made it more difficult to discuss the development of OHS without considering economic aspects. Great uncertainties in the methods employed, however, still call for caution in interpreting the results of any kind of economic appraisal. More accurate indicators, references and impact analyses are needed, and the methodological scientist faces a major challenge in this respect. It is also important to bear in mind that – in the mix of numerous economic calculations – analysis of non-monetary human health values is also needed.

Concluding remarks

The main conclusions can be summarized under the following points:

1 Financial loss from occupational injuries, diseases and lowered work ability is high, and can be roughly estimated by means of economic appraisal.
2 About one-quarter of the global disease burden is sustained by working populations. A minor part of the burden is caused directly by occupational hazards, but the overall work-related fraction is likely to be substantially higher.
3 According to recent calculations, total economic loss from occupational and work-related outcomes and lowered work ability amounts to one-sixth to one-fifth of GNP. A substantial proportion of such loss is preventable.
4 Investments in occupational health are seen to be economically profitable, or at least self-sustaining. They contribute to both loss control and increase in productivity. The establishment of OHS is, however, justified despite any such economic considerations. Productive fractions of the population need good services regardless of economic and other material values.
5 New methods for economic analysis have been developed that enable more accurate calculations of the financial consequences of occupational-health investments. Human resource analysis and ethical values are now incorporated into assessment procedures. Further methodological development, however, is still needed.

References

Aaltonen, M. (1996) A consequence and cost-analysis of occupational accidents in the furniture industry. *People and Work*. Research Reports 6. Helsinki: Finnish Institute of Occupational Health.

Ahonen, G. (1995) TERVUS-malli selvittää kannattavuuden. *Työterveiset*; **4**, 6–8 (in Finnish).

Ahonen, G. and Luopajärvi, T. (1996) *Increasing productivity and profit through health and safety. The computer program TERVUS*. Helsinki: Finnish Institute of Occupational Health.

Aronsson, T., Björk, S. and Malmquist, C. (1994) *Personalekonomi och ETIK*. Författarna och Arbetarskyddsnämnden. Stockholm: AB Grafiska Gruppen (in Swedish).

Barnum, H. (1987) Evaluating healthy days of life gained from health projects. *Soc. Sci. Med.*, **24**, 833–41.

Cooper, C.L., Liukkonen, P. and Cartwright, S. (1996) *Assessing the Benefits of Stress*

Prevention at Company Level. Dublin: European Foundation for the Improvement of Living and Working Conditions.

Hammer, J.S. (1997) Economic Analysis for Health Projects. *The World Bank Research Observer,* **1**(12), 47–71.

Hansen, S.M. (1993) *Arbejdsmiljo og samfundsokonomi – en metode til konsekvensberegning.* Nord 22. Nordisk Ministerråd (in Norwegian).

Jansson, B. and Springfeldt, B. (1996) The costs of injuries to society. In: *15 Years of Occupational Accident Research in Sweden* (E. Menckel and B. Kullinger, eds). Stockholm: Swedish Council for Work Life Research, pp. 137–48.

Koopmanschap, M.A. (1994) *Complementary Analyses in Economic Evaluation of Health Care.* Rotterdam: Erasmus University of Rotterdam.

Levi, L. and Lunde-Jensen, P. (1996) *A Model for Assessing the Costs of Stressors at National Level. Socio-economic Costs of Work Stress in two EU Member States.* Dublin: European Foundation for the Improvement of Living and Working Conditions.

Murray, C.J.L. and Lopez, A.D. (eds) (1994) *Global Comparative Assessments in the Health Sector. Disease Burden, Expenditures and Intervention Packages.* Geneva: World Health Organization.

NIOSH (National Institute for Occupational Safety and Health) (1994) *National Occupational Research Agenda.* Washington, US: NIOSH.

Rantanen, J. (1997) *Social Security Systems and Sickness Insurance – Financing and Implications in Occupational Health.* Proceedings of ICOH 4th International Conference (Scientific Committee on Health Service Research and Evaluation in Occupational Health). Rouen, April 1997 Octares, in press.

Westerholm, P. (1996) The need for legislation in occupational health services. Paper presented in International Symposium on OHS: Structure, Functions and Financing, Singapore 4–10 February (unpublished).

World Development Report. (1993) *Investing in Health.* New York: World Bank/Oxford University Press.

World Health Organization (1995) *Global Strategy on Occupational Health for All.* Geneva: World Health Organization.

21

Shifting the focus of occupational health services

Nicholas Ashford and Kathleen Rest

In this final contribution, the authors step outside the traditional frameworks for OHS evaluation that have been extensively described in this book. Adopting a broad critical perspective, they draw attention to limitations of the structure–process–outcome model. It is argued that rapid changes in the nature of work, the workforce and workplace technology impose demands for a much broader range of technical, organizational and collaborative skills on the part of OHS professionals. In particular, there is a danger that workplace technology and organization are taken as 'given'. Yet, these are the arenas in which the greatest progress is likely to be made. Although, for example, environmental and workplace demands may well conflict, it is still important to adopt a multi-dimensional approach. New evaluation approaches and metrics are required to address the inherent limitations of current production technology and work organization.

There appears to be agreement on the need for and the general objectives of occupational health services (OHS). There is also a common understanding of the range of activities, encompassing both safety and health, undertaken by OHS to achieve these objectives and on the need for an interdisciplinary OHS team. The need for OHS is based on the magnitude and burden of work-related illness, injury, disability, dysfunction and death, all of which continue to take a toll on workers, families, employers and communities throughout the industrialized and developing world. The general objectives of OHS are often based on key principles articulated by the World Health Organization and the International Labour Office. These include:

- worker protection;
- primary, secondary and tertiary prevention;
- health promotion (broadly defined);
- workplace adaptation (i.e. tailoring the work environment to the capabilities of workers);
- primary health care.

Activities that, according to van Dijk *et al.* (1993) and van der Weide *et al.* (1998), form the core of much OHS work are:

- workplace inspection;
- identification and evaluation of workplace hazards and risks;
- occupational medical services (preplacement, periodic, and incident-driven examinations);
- worker education;
- surveillance/monitoring of injury and illness in the workplace;
- consultation on sickness absence, return-to-work, and rehabilitation;
- assistance with regulatory compliance.

The growing interest in the evaluation of health care and health services in general has spilled over into occupational health care. The demand for quality, efficiency, effectiveness and acceptability of services has become more pronounced. Methods and models for evaluating health services, including OHS, have been developed and well described (Donabedian, 1988; Menckel, 1993), as too have a variety of study designs that can be used for evaluative purposes (Hulshof *et al.*, 1998; see also the chapters in this book by Øvretveit, Agius *et al.* and Verbeek *et al.*).

The complexities, methodological challenges and pitfalls that attend the evaluation of OHS have also been identified and discussed (Husman, 1993). It is clear that major stakeholders in the arena of occupational health and safety may expect different things from OHS (Draaisma, 1991; Wood *et al.*, 1987), and also that evaluations can be subject to political influences and have important political implications.

The context of the delivery and evaluation of OHS is also important and changing. OHS are designed for, and delivered at, enterprise level. The nature of work and the composition of the workforce are changing, as too are the associated 'hazards'. Such significant shifts are being accompanied by a growing interest in the application of management systems and standards to address issues of quality, quality improvement and compliance with governmental regulations (Zwetsloot and Evers, 1997). The highly competitive nature of the increasingly global economy places pressure on firms to assess their operations and eliminate those components that appear unproductive, resource depleting, or not to provide added value.

The earlier chapters in this volume provide a basis for comprehensive discussion of the theoretical and practical dimensions of evaluating OHS. For this final chapter, the editors have challenged us to step outside these frameworks and provide a broader and more critical perspective on the provision and evaluation of occupational health and safety services at enterprise level.

A critique of the current model

Implicit in the provision of OHS designed to prevent or reduce work-related injuries and diseases, and to promote worker health and well-being, is the idea that changes in inputs (resources, skills, means, etc.) followed by changes in process (interventions, activities) will result in important changes in outcomes – most often measured by the presence of hazards and resulting injuries, illnesses and disabilities. But the shortcomings and limitations of this model need to be appreciated. Efforts to evaluate the role of OHS in the prevention or reduction of occupational accidents, fatalities, injuries, diseases and disabilities (and the promotion of worker health) are confounded by many issues. Here, the following points need to be made:

- The temporal links between interventions and outcomes are sometimes long enough to obfuscate attribution of outcome to a particular intervention. When the preventable outcome is relatively rare, e.g. workplace fatalities and certain occupational diseases, the link is blurred even further.
- Some of the more prevalent work-related health problems, such as musculoskeletal disorders and stress-related illnesses, are multifactorial by nature, at times involving both workplace and non-workplace elements. The context for OHS interventions is limited to the workplace, and the traditional toolbox of the occupational safety and health professional may be better suited to monocausal problems (Rantanen, 1998).
- A host of social, economic, political and cultural factors influence many of the measures commonly used to assess 'effectiveness' or 'success' of OHS – specifically, data on absenteeism, compensation claims and injury and illness reports.
- The responsibility for workplace health and safety lies primarily with employers, who are generally free to ignore the best advice of their occupational health and safety professionals.
- The distinction between 'proximate' and 'root' causes of accidents, injuries, exposures, illnesses and disabilities is often not appreciated. Attention to proximate causes alone may do little to alter the risk of adverse outcomes. Both technology and work organization can be implicated. For example, if the root cause of a worker's musculoskeletal injury is the bad design of a tool, work process or piece of equipment, then a solution that rotates workers or enforces rest periods to decrease worker 'exposure' to the problem may simply spread the risk or postpone the injury. Similarly, if the root cause of a worker's injury is the pressure of production quotas (which led him/her to engage in an unsafe act) then a focus on the proximate cause – i.e. the worker's failure to follow written safety rules – is unlikely to prevent future injuries unless attention is also paid to production pressures (which basically invite workers to ignore safety rules in order to finish the job on time).
- Many, if not most, OHS teams accept the technology and organization of work as given. Accordingly, their recommendations for preventive interventions result in only modest changes or in easily implemented programmes, such as worker training or changes in the content and/or frequency of medical examinations. Minor tinkering with workplace technology and the organization of work may be insufficient to take us to the (next) level of injury and disease prevention and health promotion.
- The skills mix of the traditional occupational health care team may be inadequate to address the changing nature of and solutions to work-related health problems. Solutions relevant to root causes may require

technological and organizational changes that are not within the traditional knowledge base of practising health and safety professionals.

Reconceptualizing occupational health and safety practice

Workers in many small and medium-sized enterprises (SMEs) may still reap significant benefits from the delivery of traditional occupational health and safety services. Employers in SMEs need help in identifying and abating hazards, developing safety and health and return-to-work programmes, and complying with regulatory requirements. The workers in these organizations can benefit from periodic health examinations, training and education programmes, and effective therapeutic and rehabilitative services. Once accomplished, however, the probability that these traditional services will take the enterprise to the next level of injury/disease prevention and health is likely to be quite small. The next major advance in workplace health and safety will require fundamental changes in the technology and organization of the workplace. As currently configured, OHS are ill-prepared to help employers take these next steps. Yet, they will be judged on their ability to effect defined service outcomes, and will themselves suffer the economic and reputational losses if they fail to deliver improvements.

Making fundamental technological and organizational changes in the workplace demands an increased emphasis on primary prevention. Technological systems that were not designed with safety and health in mind give rise to what Charles Perrow (1984) calls 'normal accidents'. The focus of interventions in workplaces that were never designed for healthy and safer work must shift from altering human behaviour and the human–technology interface to transforming the workplace into one with 'inherently safer' technology[1] and organization.[2]

This is akin to the emphasis in the environmental field on pollution prevention or 'cleaner production'. Both cleaner production and inher-

[1] Inherent safety is an approach in chemical-accident prevention that differs fundamentally from secondary accident prevention and accident mitigation (Ashford, 1991; Kletz, 1991). 'Inherent safety' – also referred to as 'primary prevention' – relies on the development and deployment of technologies that prevent the *possibility* of a chemical accident. By comparison, 'secondary prevention' reduces the *probability* of a chemical accident, and 'mitigation' and emergency responses seek to reduce the *seriousness* of injuries, property damage and environmental damage resulting from chemical accidents. The authors are cognizant of the conventional wisdom that no technology is entirely safe. However, some technologies are in fact absolutely safe along certain dimensions. For example, some chemicals are not flammable, or explosive, or toxic. Some reactions carried out under atmospheric pressure simply will not release their byproducts in a violent way. Thus, inherent safety is analogous to pollution prevention. Like pollution prevention, the concept of inherent safety focuses attention on the proper target – the root causes of accidents and unwanted exposures.

[2] Inherently safer work organization recognizes the physical and psychosocial needs and limits of workers, designs job content and tasks to address these needs and limits and enhances the well-being of workers and does not add to the mix of risk factors that all workers carry with them into the workplace.

ently safer production call for changes in inputs (materials), production and manufacturing processes, and final products, rather than enhancements of so-called 'end-of-pipe' interventions that leave the production system and organization of work fundamentally unchanged. Making workplace technology cleaner or inherently safer will necessarily change work tasks and the organization of work. This explains, to some extent, the typical reluctance of some employers to entertain such changes. Without them, however, it may be impossible to achieve significant reductions in undesired events in the workplace.

OHS professionals can be critical agents of change in this transformation, but they must have the willingness and competence to enter the playing field. The playing field extends well beyond the traditional confines of the shopfloor and the professional consultation office, and it covers areas of business and production generally unfamiliar to the traditional health and safety team. Decisions about products, markets, production systems and methods, feedstock and other raw materials, equipment and tools (both hardware and software), work organization, size and composition of the labour force, payment systems, employee benefit packages etc. have profound effects on the health, safety and well-being of workers. Yet occupational health professionals (and workers) seldom have input into such decisions, which are seen as managerial prerogatives.[3]

OHS must expand their reach and influence into all areas of the organization that can affect worker health and safety. This will require an expanded team of professionals, and also enhanced competence among traditional team members in certain areas. To advance the cause of cleaner and inherently safer technology, OHS will need to acquire expertise in materials science, process, mechanical and biomechanical engineering, synthetic organic chemistry, and toxicology. The creation of 'inherently healthier and safer' work organizations will require expertise in human and industrial psychology, sociology, human physiology, human factors, labour relations, and organizational change.

In addition to these skills, the ability to understand and appreciate the production or service-delivery demands on employers struggling to compete in the new global market is critical to persuading reluctant or sceptical employers to integrate health and safety concerns into all aspects of the enterprise. A knowledge of economics, quality and resource management, cost accounting and legal obligations are essential for meaningful interactions with firm managers and owners. As the first president of the European Network of Societies of Occupational Physicians (ENSOP) stated at the organization's first General Assembly Meeting in June 1998, occupational physicians [and, we would argue, other members of an expanded occupational health care team], must leave the safety of their consulting rooms, learn to speak the language of enterprise managers, and be bold enough to enter the boardrooms of organi-

---

[3]For an argument that workers ought to be able to bargain with management over technological changes that affect their health and safety, see Chapter 7 in Ashford and Caldart (1996).

zations to argue for the changes needed to create safe and healthy workplaces (van der Vliet, 1998).

Beyond the acquisition of new skills, there is an urgent need for OHS professionals to work together. This is because a focus on root causes of accidents, exposures, injuries and illnesses could lead to fundamental changes in production technology that potentially address and solve a host of problems faced by an enterprise. For example, fundamental redesign of a cutting machine could have positive impacts on noise levels (and noise-induced hearing loss), vibration (and upper-extremity musculoskeletal problems), machine–human interactions (and strains, sprains, lacerations, and abrasions), environmental waste (by changing the nature and/or volume of cutting fluids), and product quality (through enhanced precision of the cutting operation). If concerns for health, safety environment and product quality can be integrated and addressed simultaneously by a solution posed by an OHS team, the likelihood that the enterprise will make the necessary investment is greater.

Towards a new approach to evaluating OHS

What does all this portend for the critical issue of evaluation? It places a heavy burden on those who provide and those who evaluate OHS. Not only must they attend to the challenges and confounders discussed early in this chapter, they must also identify and rationalize new dimensions for evaluation. This book has offered practical guidance on how to address some of the methodological problems involved in evaluating occupational health and safety services and interventions, implicitly focusing on the workplace as more-or-less given and fundamentally unchangeable. Within this framework, some of the limitations of evalua-tion methodologies can be addressed. For example, it is important to allow sufficient time for interventions to show an effect. For some outcomes – rare events (such as fatalities), long-latency diseases and conditions that are multifactorial by nature – it may be inappropriate to use changes in the health outcomes themselves as measures of success. In these cases, it is more appropriate to focus on process variables and outcome measures that relate to hazard reduction/elimination – or the extent to which the technology is made cleaner or inherently safer.

By contrast, addressing the inherent limitations of current production technology and work organization requires additional and different evaluation approaches and metrics. New outcome measures may include such things as the substitution of safer and less toxic materials, safer and cleaner manufacturing, production and service-delivery processes, more satisfying and humane jobs, work tasks and work organization, different ways of delivering services, more human-friendly (anthropocentric) work environments, evolution of organizations that learn and continu-ously improve (to name just a few).

In sum, while the model of structure, process and outcome evaluation discussed throughout this volume will continue to have merit, the components of these parameters will have to be expanded to encompass the newly conceptualized occupational health and safety practice. Development and use of suitable evaluation metrics will be the next challenge.

A final note. While changes to production-manufacturing and service-delivery technologies, and also work organization, hold the promise of injury/disease prevention and health promotion, changes in technology are already being influenced by environmental demands. Unfortunately, professionals and regulatory agencies concerned with the environment often do not consider or coordinate their efforts with worker health and safety (and vice-versa). Moreover, the environment has a higher priority on the agenda of most industrialized economies. There is already evidence that pollution-prevention technologies may inadvertently either exacerbate the health and safety problems of workers or miss opportunities to make things better (Ashford et al., 1996; Ashford, 1997). This tendency underscores the necessity for environmental and OHS professionals to work together to design technologies that are both environmentally and workplace sound.

References

Ashford, N.A. (1991) Policy considerations for anticipating and preventing accidents. *Proceedings of Enprotech '91 International Environmental Conference*, Taiwan, 30–31 January 1991.

Ashford, N.A. (1997) Industrial safety: the neglected issue in industrial ecology. In: Special Issue on Industrial Ecology (N.A. Ashford and R.P. Côté, eds). *J. Cleaner Production*, **5**(1/2), 115–21.

Ashford, N., Banoutsos, I., Christiansen, K., Hummelmose, B. and Stratikopoulos, D. (1996) *Evaluation of the Relevance for Worker Health and Safety of Existing Environmental Technology Data-bases for Cleaner and Inherently Safer Technologies: A Report to the European Commission*, April 1996.

Ashford, N.A. and Caldart, C.C. (1996) *Technology, Law and the Working Environment*, 2nd edn. Washington, DC: Island Press.

Donabedian, A. (1988) The quality of care. How can it be assessed? *JAMA*, **260**, 1743–8.

Draaisma, D., de Winter, C.R., Dam, J., van den Heuvel, S.G. (1991) *Quality and Effectiveness of Occupational Health Care*. The Hague: Ministry of Social Affairs and Employment (in Dutch).

Hulshof, C.T.J., Verbeek, J.H.A.M., van Dijk, F.J.H., van der Weide, W.E. and Braam, I.T.J. (1998) Evaluation research in OHS. General principles and a model of OHS evaluation. In: *Prevention and Control of Adverse Effects of Whole-Body Vibration: An Evaluation Study in OHS* (C.T.J. Hulshof, ed.) Academic Thesis, University of Amsterdam.

Husman, K. (1993) Principles and pitfalls in health services research in occupational health systems. *Occup. Med.*, **43** (Suppl 1), S10–14.

Kletz, T.A. (1991) *Plant Design for Safety*. New York: Hemisphere Publishing.

Menckel, E. (1993) *Evaluating and Promoting Change in OHS – Models and Applications*. Stockholm: The Swedish Work Environment Fund.

Perrow, C. (1984) *Normal Accidents: Living with High-risk Technologies*. New York: Basic Books.

Rantanen, J. (1998) OHS in the prevention of work-related diseases. Paper presented at *PREMUS-ISEOH '98 Conference*, 21–25 September 1998, Helsinki, Finland.

van Dijk, F.J.H., de Kort, W. and Verbeek, J.H.A.M. (1993) Quality assessment of occupational health services. *Occup. Med.*, **43**(supp. 1), 28–33.

van der Vliet, J.A. (1988) Challenges for the future. Presentation at the First General Assembly Meeting of ENSOP, Brussels, 12 June 1998.

van der Weide, W., Verbeek, J., van Dijk, F. and Hulshof, C. (1998) Development and evaluation of a quality assessment instrument for occupational physicians. *Occupational and Environmental Medicine*, **55**, 375–382.

Wood, J.M., Kelman, R., Pilkington, W., Patfield, S., Walker, G. and Harrison A. (1987) Comparative perceptions of the delivery of OHS in industry. *J. Occup. Hlth Safety Aust NZ*, **3**, 632–8.

Zwetsloot, G. and Evers, G. (1997) The added value of total health and safety management. In: *Costs and Benefits of Occupational Safety and Health. Proceedings of the European Conference on Costs and Benefits of Occupational Safety and Health 1997* (J. Mossink and F. Licher, eds). The Hague, 28–30 May 1997, Amsterdam: NIA–TNO.

Index